How
Broccoli-Head
Lost
Thirty Pounds

A HANDBOOK TO HEALTHY LIVING

Anselm Anyoha, MD

iUniverse, Inc.
Bloomington

HOW BROCCOLI-HEAD LOST THIRTY POUNDS
A HANDBOOK TO HEALTHY LIVING

iUniverse books may be ordered through booksellers or by contacting:

iUniverse
1663 Liberty Drive
Bloomington, IN 47403
www.iuniverse.com
1-800-Authors (1-800-288-4677)

ISBN: 978-1-4759-8757-7 (sc)
ISBN: 978-1-4759-8759-1 (hc)
ISBN: 978-1-4759-8758-4 (e)

Library of Congress Control Number: 2013907397

Printed in the United States of America.

iUniverse rev. date: 5/22/2013

To my children and my family, who had to grapple with my new, trim look; and to my amazing patients, who continue to inspire and challenge me to provide more quality health care. Especially to my wife, Sandra Nneka, who nicknamed me "Broccoli-Head" after I ate so much broccoli that she could smell it in my hair.

Disclaimer

The book is not meant to diagnose or treat any conditions. Every attempt was made to include only accurate information, but the author absolves himself of any factual error of omission or commission. Readers must do their own due diligence in checking out all materials presented in this book and also consult with their physicians before trying any recommendations in this book. The book was based on the author's experience and perspective and may not be suitable for all.

Contents

Preface

I embarked on this book because lots of my friends, family, and patients wanted to know my method for losing thirty pounds and how I was able to sustain my current weight of 152–154 pounds for nearly twenty-four months.

In formulating an answer, I discovered many things that I did not know about food and health. I want to share this information with the readers of this book.

Since losing thirty pounds, I have completed one book and am finishing this book. I attribute the resurgence of my creative energy to my physical fitness. I am ecstatic. My body has stopped craving junk food at every gas station and minimarket stop.

It is not hard to understand why one should eat healthy food and exercise regularly. The difficulty is in doing it and making that choice a lifelong habit. We need to understand the dynamics between our health and the food and drink we consume. Obstacles to achieving a healthy lifestyle are numerous, and the consequences are very costly in terms of money and quality of life.

Before writing this book, I was like many practicing physicians—ignorant of the basic tenets of nutrition. Many people also seem unaware that the surest way to put on weight is to go on an added-sugar binge.

Good advice on healthy eating—an important subject—has been buried under the greed and commercialization of food producers. This book reaches out from under the current fad-food and fitness mania to offer salient and lifesaving information to the general public.

Weight, food, nutrition, and diet are subjects that can be discussed on multiple levels. This book brings all these dimensions under one umbrella.

The fight to lose weight must be addressed by eating nature's food and exercising. When we eat healthy, plant-based food, we align ourselves with the vibrancy of nature. Exercise makes the body's processing machinery quick and animated.

Though this book is devoted to nutrition and healthy weight, as well as obesity as a factor in disease propagation and health management, readers must understand that not every overweight or obese person has a health concern. Likewise, many diseases develop without there being a weight issue.

Food provides the energy needed for the cells to function, but food in excess of what the body needs can smother cellular machinery and cause dysfunction.

I was motivated to write this book based on my own experience and success. I didn't purchase any "get fit" tapes, and I didn't subscribe to a ready-to-eat food plan. I didn't join a gym or fitness center, and I didn't purchase exercise equipment to use at home. All I needed was my old gym pants that I dusted off from the back of my closet and a basketball that I inflated after I salvaged it from my garage. Then, I simply ate appropriately and exercised.

Before you waste money on gym memberships or prepackaged food plans, try to gain the proper insight into the weight dilemma. Use this book as a manual on your weight-loss journey and a guide and reminder during a weight-gain relapse.

Introduction

Y ou may have read other books about weight loss, healthy food, fitness, and dieting, but you are about to read a book that was written by a middle-aged doctor who actually lost thirty pounds and has maintained it, as of this writing, for two years. I am my own testimony. What I did was simple, and it worked. I'll bet it will work for you.

CHAPTER 1

My Story and Body Profile

Many times, it is a particular event in our lives that stops our wavering on what we need to do and jolts us into resolute actions. For me, it was a visit to my primary care physician for an annual physical exam. I only went because it was mandated by the hospital where I had privileges—if I didn't get an annual exam, my hospital privileges would not be renewed. I felt fine, though, and continued to perform my daily routine of seeing patients and prescribing drugs. Suddenly, however, I was going to be a patient.

Switching from being the healer to being the afflicted was not only a humbling experience, but it also imparted a perspective I rarely see. This wasn't my first time as a patient, of course, but this time I dwelled on the patient/physician dynamics. Foremost in my mind was wondering how knowledgeable my doctor would be and how invested he would be in making sure that I got the best advice and treatment available. Fortunately, the doctor who took my blood pressure was a friend, someone I know to be very conscientious, knowledgeable, and successful in the practice of medicine. Patients wait for hours to see him, sometimes camping out in the hallway because the waiting room cannot accommodate everyone.

The results of my physical exam indicated that my blood pressure had gone up to 140/90 and that my LDL (low-density lipoprotein, the "bad" cholesterol) had also increased. These numbers meant that I was mildly hypertensive and had an abnormally high level of LDL.

Hypertension, or high blood pressure, is when a person's blood pressure exceeds 140 mm of mercury in the upper number (called systolic value) and/or exceeds 90 in the lower number, the diastolic value. Depending on the measured number, hypertension is classified as mild, moderate, severe, or malignant.

Hypertension can occur for a number of reasons. Obesity is one of the well-known but preventable and reversible causes of high blood pressure. At the office visit, my weight was 183 pounds, and I am five foot seven. At first glance, a weight of 183 pounds does not sound excessive, but taking my height into consideration, my BMI showed I was overweight by a whopping thirty pounds. Had my doctor been interested in nutrition or paid attention to the connection between excessive weight and high blood pressure, his advice to me would have been to go home, work out my weight issue, and come back at a later date for a blood pressure recheck. He missed that opportunity, however, and instead, he offered me a pill to bring down my blood pressure.

My predicament was not unusual, and my doctor's favored solution of prescribing pills was not an exception. Many people don't realize they have high blood pressure. If they are lucky, like I was, they are diagnosed during a routine office visit. If they are unlucky, like so many people with no access to primary care doctors, their high blood pressure is discovered only when it is complicated by a stroke or kidney disease or it compromises their heart function.

Dealing effectively with obesity-related high blood pressure requires a multifaceted approach and dedication by the physician and the patient, both of whom have vital roles to play in this management. Unfortunately, many practicing physicians find it easier and more cost effective to quickly prescribe a medication rather than counsel a solution. The link between obesity and hypertension and so many other diseases is not foremost in physicians' thoughts. Furthermore, many patients are not receptive to any solution other than a quick fix.

At the end of my visit, the doctor offered his solution: he would prescribe a daily dose of chlorothiazides (a diuretic). "I have a similar problem," he confided, "and have been taking a stronger version of the same medicine for years."

He was persuasive, but I declined to follow his example. I opted out for two reasons: First, taking medication for what seemed to be obesity-related high blood pressure was similar to covering a wound with a Band-Aid. The Band-Aid does not make the wound go away. One must tackle the underlying cause of the problem. Second, his recommendation did not sit well with me when I considered some of the side effects associated with chlorothiazides. These include liver or kidney impairment, heart rhythm disturbances, high blood-sugar level, potential for diabetes, disturbance of blood lipid levels, nausea, vomiting, and sodium- and potassium-balance disruption.

At the back of my mind was an escape route; it led to giving in to the challenges of life and acquiescing to society's expectation, which is for middle-aged folks to quickly transition to old age, infirmity, and eternity. Fortunately, I realized that was a dead end; it's a path I hope no one will elect.

I was close to age fifty at this time, and my options seemed limited. Exercise might help control my blood pressure, but I did not have the energy for intense workouts. I knew I needed to change my lifestyle, but how could I relearn good behaviors that I had abandoned long ago?

I knew about the relationship between weight and blood pressure. The more I learned about that relationship, the more I was determined to fix my elevated blood pressure the right way—by losing weight. And that is what I did. I went and had my last bacon, egg, and cheese on a toasted croissant, cut down on my calories, and switched to nature's own food.

Below is a summary of my initial actions.

Quick fix: Replace old bad habits with new good habits.

Old habits	New habit
Extra night job	Switch to extra day job
Breakfast: fried egg sandwich with butter, cheese, any bread, coffee with sugar	Boiled egg sandwich, whole-grain bread, coffee, no sugar please

Morning snack: cookies, cashew nuts	Grapes and salads
Lunch: bacon, egg, and cheese on croissant	Oatmeal and steamed vegetable, or baked potato, or whole legumes and grains
Afternoon snack: more cookies and nuts	None, or more salads
Dinner: fried plantain and egg	Vegetable soup, beans, lentils, peas
Food as an escape route	Exercise as an escape route
Holiday as an excuse to binge	Holiday as an excuse to eat healthily
Constipated	Bowel movement
Beer and soda	Water and water
Eat at a set time	Eat when hungry
Acquiesce to junk food	Say no to junk food
Blind to food labels	Aware of food label, including details of food description
Eat out	Eat at home
French fries for dessert	No French fries
Ate whatever was on my plate	Tell people exactly what I do not want in my food
Their recipe	My recipe

The result was a thirty-pound weight loss in three months and a blood pressure reading of 110/70. My weight has remained around 150 pounds for two years and counting.

Achieving what I wished for took a lot of hard work and commitment. Like many people, I had my share of daily stress and scheduling conflicts. Finding a way to squeeze my weight-burden task into my professional and family responsibilities was a balancing act that required tact and judgment.

Not many careers are as demanding as private medical practice. My daily wake-up time is early. By six thirty, I am in my office to complete my clinical notes and other paperwork. Office hours start at 9:00 a.m. and end at 6:30 p.m. By the time I get home, it is between seven and eight. Then it's time for the kids, dealing with their growing pains and school issues.

Prior to my physical exam, I knew that I was not eating right and hadn't exercised for a long time. By the end of the day, there was hardly any time left for personal care. So the brief look at my health status was a wake-up call.

But how could I have possibly veered so far away from my nutritional upbringing? Junk food was hardly on my menu as a young boy growing up in the urban city of Onitsha, Nigeria. My mother cooked. We ate grains, yam, cassava, and vegetables. In the villages where we lived, we played soccer all day and plucked from every fruit-bearing tree. Eating junk food was a habit I developed when I came to the United States. I had never seen French fries until I got to the subways of New York City. My first cup of coffee was probably at age thirty-two when I began my residency training program at Brookdale Hospital in Brooklyn, New York. With caffeine in my bloodstream, I could stay up during medical night calls. Then, of course, the pressure of time and stress meant that I had to continue with the fast pace and the fast food. Well, if I had learned to eat junk, I could learn to reverse that habit and eat nature's own food. Like hypertension, several other diseases are linked to excessive weight gain and obesity, including gall bladder disease, coronary artery disease, stroke, and diabetes.

The gains are definitely worth the effort. I have not suffered from flu for two consecutive years. I've had no symptoms of my former seasonal allergies in two years. My hair, though graying, is lustrous and thick. My abdominal girth is flat. I can outlast many teens in physical endurance. The time spent in caring for personal well-being is a value investment, today and for the future, and I am ecstatic.

Quitting junk food was easy to do. Once my mind was made up, I dumped the usual suspects: fried chicken, fried potatoes, doughnuts, flavored milk or sugar for coffee, French fries, sodas, beer, fried plantains, and chocolates. Surprisingly, I did not miss any of it after a week or so.

In addition to abandoning unhealthy food, I also started exercising. I set up specific time for exercises and stuck to it. I used the neighborhood high school track field, the local parks, and the town gym. I walked the trails, shot basketballs, and ran up the hills and stairs. The weight began to peel off. Success begot success, and I was able to continue these activities until I lost thirty pounds.

Initially, I relied on common sense and knowledge and ate only what felt right. I did that because at first I wanted to discover what worked for me in my own experience, making my own mistakes and adjustments, rather than listening to someone else's opinion. Eventually, I did research other people's understanding of nutrition and tapped into their collective knowledge. I was ready to learn what people who had similar concerns did. During my research, I discovered why the obesity epidemic has taken over about half of the entire population of the United States and the world. I also stumbled into a world of food and nutrients that I had not known existed. My triumphant story of weight loss is based on my reminding myself why I began this journey and why it is necessary to continue.

CHAPTER 2

The Obesity Epidemic

Obesity does not respect class—rich, poor, or middle class, anyone can be obese, although often for different reasons. Some people may be obese because of the abundance of food at their disposal, while others may be overweight because of restrictive or poor choices of food.

The obesity epidemic in the United States and elsewhere in the world can be attributed to two broad reasons: overconsumption of food and less physical activity. People are finding more reasons to eat big meals, yet fewer reasons to break a sweat. Restaurants and fast-food outlets are under competitive pressure to increase the size of the food portions and beverages they serve. From hamburgers to pizza to pasta, the size of individual portions has skyrocketed exponentially.

Recently, I took my family out to eat at a local restaurant. I ordered a kid's portion for my twelve-year-old son, but when his meal came, it looked like enough to fill two full-grown, hungry men. I asked the waitress, "Is this the kid's size we ordered?" She assured me it was. I watched my son struggle to finish the meal. I could tell he was full after eating one-fourth, because after that he paused many times while eating to catch his breath. I wouldn't have minded as much if he'd been eating a bowl of steamed broccoli and spinach, but it was macaroni and cheese.

Availability of food

Easy access to food outlets leads to constant purchase and consumption of food. For example, you not only can get coffee, snacks, and doughnuts not only from grocery stores but also from gas stations or fitness centers, and from vending machines in hospital lobbies, banks, or on street corners. Many stores are now multitasking—pharmacies not only dispense drugs but also nuts, crackers, and cookies. Food and snacks constantly are in our faces. And with that comes the temptation to eat.

Food as a companion

Many of us eat or drink out of habit—not because we are hungry or thirsty at the moment but because we feel an urge to do something in addition to the task at hand. Food serves as convenient glue to connect our sets of activities. Food is frequently used to fill the void whenever we have to wait. A late bus or train or plane gives us an excuse to dash across the lobby to purchase a snack or drink or another cup of tea with sugar. We bring food along as a companion on trips. Why do we find it difficult to concentrate on the task at hand? Think about what would happen if a surgeon reached for a snack while removing someone's appendix.

Food advertisements and cost

Whoever controls the airwaves often controls the message. Big food outlets have the capacity to advertise their business and lure people to patronize them, so they strategically control a substantial part of what we buy or eat. They bombard television and radio, targeting children's and adults' favorite programs as the time to market their food, which often is processed food. For unclear reasons, healthy and natural produce tends to be costlier than processed food. It could be that processed foods are cheaper to produce, while healthy produce takes a lot more human involvement and is more difficult to produce. In the end, the cost of production, which is high for healthy food, is passed along to the consumer, while the savings in production, which is low for processed foods, benefits those who eat junk.

Social/cultural behavior

People tend to eat more during social events. The proliferation of holidays—national, religious, and ethnic—has given people the opportunity to engage in excessive eating and drinking. From Thanksgiving celebrations to Christmas, to Hanukkah, to President's Day, to Veteran's Day, to Kwanza, it is all party time. And there are people who have social engagements every weekend throughout the year. Society, it seems, has accepted it as the norm to pair food with holidays, to the extent that a person may be considered odd if he or she opts out of the holiday food frenzy.

In what I have termed "event-food syndrome," people tend to plunge headlong into food gluttony as a way to celebrate—their minds have been taken over by food at that moment. They use any occasion to devour all the processed, sweetened food they can find. These are the people who tend to gain back lost weight rapidly, because they have not resolved why they needed to diet or eat healthily.

Whether you are the host or hostess who serves the food or the guest to whom the food is offered, the food of choice is probably sweet and tasty. People expect to be fed and treated to cake, ice cream, hot dogs, soda or Kool-Aid, and chips. This is the way it has always been, and it is very difficult to overcome that expectation. Today's society, more than in any other time, associates social occasions with eating and drinking.

Culture sometimes plays a part in obesity, as in some cultures, a large body size is considered a sign of wealth and well-being. A lean body is regarded as a sign of poverty. Some kids and adults are cajoled to keep eating, even when they are no longer hungry.

Stress/lack of awareness

Food is sometimes used as an escape route for stress and boredom. Some of us eat as a way to compensate for the emotional turmoil of stress.

There is increasing stress in America and the developing world. Stress often is related to our jobs or income. When we worry about how we will make it to the next paycheck, we may reach for more snacks and other food as a way to soothe ourselves.

Many people still do not appreciate the relationship between junk food, sugary beverages, and obesity. While counseling a teenager on her weight, I learned that the youngster drank a lot of Kool-Aid. When I inquired why, her mother's answer jolted me: "Because packs of powdered Kool-Aid are usually on sale."

Food phobia

Food phobia is a tendency for some people to eat only a particular food or from a particular food group—for example, someone may eat only macaroni and cheese, or cheeseburgers, or any other single food item. Eating one food group not only limits the body's exposure to nutrients available in the neglected food but also could be a gateway to obesity, especially if the favored food is high in calories and fat.

Night-shift workers

People who work the night shift tend to eat during late hours at work. Our body metabolism tends to be somewhat dormant during late-night hours, and this habit may lead to weight gain. In addition, people who work the night shift may mistake body fatigue as hunger and indulge in frequent snacking.

Time constraints

Time is an issue that compounds obesity. People increasingly spend less time at home and more time trying to earn money, which means less time to prepare their own meals, leaving them vulnerable to eating fast food and meals prepared outside the home. The problem with eating out is that we must rely on someone else to prepare our meals, and those meals are often loaded with salt or sugar. The same people who lack time to prepare a healthy meal at home often lack the time for any physical activities.

Time that could be allotted to physical activities usually conflicts with other equally important time-demanding tasks, such as child care, school activities, social engagements, or care of elderly parents. Feeling socially isolated also can be a hindrance to physical activities. This feeling may be exaggerated when an individual or family moves to a new location.

Disease and disability

Any disease condition resulting in poor body metabolism or slow mobility may predispose an individual to excessive weight gain. Low-functioning thyroid glands, hypothyroidism, or neuromuscular diseases such as Duchenne muscular dystrophy are just a few of such conditions. Genetic disorders such as Prader-Willi syndrome can cause, among other symptoms, an irresistible urge to eat, which will result in weight gain. Athletes' use of steroids to reach a certain weight requirement or to gain a certain competitive advantage is a growing cause of excessive weight gain and obesity.

Circumstances associated with decreased mobility, such as illness, can dramatically cut down on a person's physical activity level and lead to weight gain, especially if the caloric intake remains the same or is increased. People on steroids for chronic medical illness also accumulate fluid and gain weight. People who experience shortness of breath during exercise are limited in their capacity to do so. People with bone issues, such as arthritis or a slipped disc, could also be limited in their exercise capacity. These conditions must be checked out and be properly diagnosed by well-qualified clinicians before engaging in physical activities.

Love

Ever wonder why people put on weight after they get married? They are following the supposition that the surest "way to a man's heart is through his stomach." The setup for this starts at the wedding reception, when couples stuff each other's mouth with cake. Then it continues through the honeymoon and afterward. One must eat to show one's love to one's spouse, whether or not one likes the food or is hungry.

I attended an event where we were served a full-course meal with dessert. Everybody was full to throat level. You might think that everyone was eager to get home and sleep, but one guy said to me, "No matter how full I am, I always eat when I get home." When I asked him why he would eat again if he was full, he responded, "My wife will be unhappy if I don't eat her home-cooked food."

Type of food/activity

The type of food we eat is of tremendous importance. Eating fast food and processed food is a sure way to put on weight. Salty food, sugary food, and fried food also can cause weight gain and should not be a part of a regular, healthy diet. In addition to the type of food, however, obesity also can be the result of diminished physical activities.

Some people lose interest in physical activity as they get older. They may think that physical activities are for kids, who need to keep busy to stay out of trouble. That is good, but older people also need to be physically engaged. It is troubling to see an overweight parent or caregiver taking a fit child to a sports activity. Why don't the adults take time to be physically fit as well? Just because someone turns forty, gets married, has a child or two, works long hours doesn't mean he or she should jettison physical activities.

There is a vital relationship between how heavy we are and our activity level. Even if our calorie intake remains the same as we get older, a decrease in physical activity will cause us to put on weight. Therefore, we must maintain our activity level or cut our daily caloric intake as we get older in order to maintain a healthy weight.

It does take time, however, so don't think you can easily burn up all of the calories you accumulated in seven minutes of gluttony. It is much easier to gain weight than to lose it.

Accessibility

Accessibility may be a factor in a lack of physical activity. There may be no safe locations for one to exercise or work out in the immediate neighborhood. If you live in an apartment and work out at home, neighbors might complain about the noise associated with a workout.

Winter presents a unique constraint for some people. They may not like to exercise outdoors in cold weather, particularly if the ground is covered with snow. Indoor facilities are often more crowded in winter, with people competing to use the equipment. On three occasions in January, I drove to the town's fitness center but could not find an available spot for my basketball activities. The court was occupied by kids.

Body type and weight

Propensity to gain weight and slow metabolism may be related to body types. The differences between individual body shapes are mostly determined genetically by the underlying skeletal anatomy, as well as somewhat by the overlying fat pad. Some of us have broad shoulders, for example, while others have narrow shoulders. The three main categories to human body shape include:

- **Ectomorph**
  Ectomorphs possess a narrow frame or cylindrical body shape. Fat does not seem to stick on them, at least not for very long. These people will tell you that everybody in their family is thin. They are blessed with a high metabolism.

- **Mesomorph**
  Mesomorphs have the V-shaped body of broad shoulders, broad chest, and narrow trunk and waist. Mesomorphs have an average metabolism but usually have little issue with retaining fat, although it may be more of an issue than it is for ectomorphs.

- **Endomorph**
  Endomorphs' bodies are plump and round—a magnet for fat and weight gain. Everything they eat seems to stick on them. They may have inherited a sluggish metabolism.

CHAPTER 3

Signs of Obesity and Associated Diseases

It is easy to spot someone who is grossly overweight; technically speaking, one is overweight when his or her body mass index (BMI) is greater than 24.9. A person is considered obese when his or her BMI exceeds 30. Low energy, lack of stamina, inability to keep pace with ordinary activities, and/or exercise intolerance are usual complaints of overweight and obese people.

For every visibly obese person, there are many others who are grossly overweight but have fallen through the cracks of societal observation. Common external signs of being overweight and obesity are fat cells that invade and occupy all parts of the body.

Your body type has a limit to its ability to guard you against weight gain. Fat is a versatile molecule, capable of organizing and colonizing any part of the body. If you do not eat properly, fat will overwhelm you and appear in your cheeks, your neck, your chest, your legs, your butt, and your belly. Excess fat deposits in the face and around the cheeks give a rounded "baby face," like a cherub. Once you get your nutrition and exercise under control, the fat around the face will dissolve along with overall general body fat.

I once asked a woman who had a protruding abdomen when her baby was due. I was deeply embarrassed to learn she was not pregnant. Excluding any true medical condition, abdominal protrusion, or pot belly, is due to fat accumulation in the abdominal muscle. Similarly, fat can accumulate in the legs, back of the neck, chest, buttocks, and hands.

Fat stretch marks, called *striae*, may appear on the skin due to rapid weight gain. These marks, normally seen over the abdomen during pregnancy, are also visible on people who are overweight or obese.

Rough skin or a rash caused by friction of the inner thighs is frequently seen in overweight people, as oversized thighs rub together.

Acanthosis nigricans is a term that refers to the dark pigmentation, mostly at the nape of the neck or the elbows, that usually is seen in individuals who are obese or overweight. It could be an external sign of insulin resistance and prediabetes.

Fat is motile—it can invade any body organs. One of the most recognizable signs of such a condition is when wayward fat tissues infiltrate the liver, causing what is now widely known as the nonalcoholic fatty liver disease. Accumulation of fat in liver cells may lead to inflammation or disruption and dysfunction of the liver. Obesity is one of many conditions that predispose one to fatty liver formation.

Not only does fat produce visible, gross body effects, but it also contributes to numerous medical conditions, including the following:

- hypertension
- diabetes
- degenerative arthritis
- depression
- cancer
- gout
- stroke
- ischemic heart disease
- gallstones
- sleep apnea

Some of the above-listed diseases associated with obesity and overweight are discussed below. Please note that these diseases are not restricted to those people who are obese or overweight, nor does everyone who is obese or overweight necessarily have these conditions.

Sleep apnea

Sleep apnea is an abnormal cessation or compromise of breathing that occurs during sleep. A person's flow of oxygen from the nostril or mouth through the windpipe to the lung is compromised because of obstruction within the upper airway channels. Breathing is an involuntary phenomenon, but people often become aware of their breathing mechanism if they breathe with some effort, such as when the nostrils are congested during a cold or flu.

Sleep apnea is a serious problem because it occurs when consciousness is low, and so the ability to exert breathing effort also is low. Oxygenation of blood is poor during sleep apnea.

People with inadequate oxygen delivery to the lungs and blood as a result of sleep apnea seldom sleep well at night. They wake up frequently during sleep, and they toss and turn as they gasp for air and fight to breathe. Attempts to overcome the obstruction in breathing may result in loud snoring or chest wall and neck muscle retractions. The consequence, which is a poor night's sleep, translates to daytime fatigue.

The exact manner in which obesity causes sleep apnea is not totally clear, but some theories include:

- The weight of fat around the windpipe causes it to collapse and obstruct breathing.
- It's a result of blunted reflexes around the upper airways or respiratory channels, which can be associated with the various fat tissues' hormonal and neuronal abnormalities.

Other diseases must be considered and investigated before the diagnosis of obesity-associated sleep apnea can be definitively made. In general, weight loss helps ameliorate some of the signs and symptoms of obesity-associated apnea.

Gallstones

The gallbladder is an organ located under the liver that stores bile, a fluid made by the liver to digest fat. Gallbladder disease is commonly seen in middle-aged, overweight females, but it can occur in both sexes and even in adolescents. Two types of gallstones may develop in the gallbladder—cholesterol gallstones, which account for the majority of the gallstones, and pigmented gallstones, which account for about a quarter of all cases.

The bile produced and stored in the liver is necessary, among other things, for the digestion of fat in the meals we eat. For some reason, stones frequently develop in this "bile soup" before it is deployed for fat digestion.

Probable reasons for gallstone formation include:

- high cholesterol content in bile
- gallbladder dysfunction, as result of hormones or cytokines produced by fat tissues
- obesity, which leads to bile instability and stone formation

Once formed, gallstones can dislodge from the gallbladder to any part of the biliary anatomical system, where they cause conduit blockage, pain, and infection. For example, the blockage of the pancreatic duct where it joins the biliary system causes inflammation of the pancreas, known as pancreatitis. The pancreas is an important organ because its cells produces insulin, which is essential in the control of blood glucose.

People may harbor stones in their gallbladders without realizing it. Only a third of the people with gallstones will develop signs and symptoms. One of the commonest symptoms of gallstones includes recurrent pain in the upper right side of the abdomen. Pain can radiate to the right shoulder. Aversion to fatty foods, abdominal bloating, and flatulence can also be symptoms associated with gallstones.

If not treated or recognized early, complications can occur, resulting in deterioration of the gallbladder and manifesting as fever and a yellowish tinge in the white part of the eyes (jaundice). Life-threatening infection and death can occur due to *choledocholithiasis*, which refers to the presence of one or more gallstones obstructing the very important common bile duct.

Diagnosis of gallstones is mostly through a specialized imaging technique using ultrasound. Treatment may include surgical removal of gallstones or *cholecystectomy*, the surgical removal of the gallbladder. Half a million such surgeries, costing close to five billion dollars annually, are performed in the United States.

Hypertension

Blood pressure refers to the pressure exerted in the arteries (the systemic vasculature) as blood is pumped out from the heart and to the rest of the body. The circulatory system vasculatures can be likened to a system of tubes with varying sizes, calibers, and thicknesses. The amount of pressure exerted by blood flow on a blood vessel is influenced by how rapid the heart is beating, the size of the particular vessel, how far it is from the heart, and the internal resistance of the vasculature.

There are two numbers to remember when talking about high blood pressure. The top number—the systolic reading—measures the blood pressure when the heart is pumping blood, and the bottom number—the diastolic blood pressure reading—measures the blood pressure when the heart is relaxing and not in active pumping mode. Readings above 140/90 are abnormal in adult age groups. (Numbers for children are different.)

High blood pressure is harmful to the human body, especially to the kidneys, where it can injure the filtration units, called the nephrons. It is also damaging to the heart, where it can lead to weak heart muscles and heart failure. It is also harmful to the brain, where it can lead to vasculature rupture and strokes.

How obesity causes high blood pressure

Fat tissue in the body acts as exocrine cells to produce hormone-like substances, sometimes called adipokines, that are capable of elevating systemic blood pressure by increasing sympathetic drive and vascular tone.

Another way in which obesity can cause high blood pressure is by upsetting the normal self-feedback mechanism that the body has to get rid of its excessive salt and water. This pathway is called the renin, aldosterone, and angiotensin mechanism. Also, the condition of high insulin secretion, insulin resistance, and insensitivity seen in obesity predisposes the body to salt or sodium retention, which contributes to high blood pressure.

Heart attack and coronary artery disease

Chest pain is one of the most dreaded symptoms, because chest pain can be a sign of ischemic heart disease, a condition where blood supply to heart muscles, which are required to pump blood to all parts of the body, has been compromised. The human heart is a hollowed, pumping muscle. The hard-working muscles of the heart need to be well supplied with oxygenated blood in other to retain the power to pump blood for the entire body.

What can cause occlusion of the blood supply to heart muscles? Very often, it is lipoproteins, which are made of protein and fat, from which a coronary artery vasculature occlusion develops. *Lipoproteins* are compounds normally found in the blood that transport fat across cell membranes into the blood vessels. Lipoproteins occur in different sizes and forms, but for the purpose of this discussion, we will focus on low density lipoprotein (LDL) and the high density lipoprotein (HDL).

LDL is thought to be deleterious to the vasculatures that supply blood, oxygen, and nutrients to the heart muscle and blood vessels and therefore need to be regularly cleared and gotten rid of by the high-density counterpart, HDL.

Failure of HDL to clear LDL will result in the accumulation of LDL. Buildup of LDL damages the walls of blood vessels supplying the heart muscle and other vital parts of the heart. Soon thereafter, an inflammation ensues around the damaged area with most of the inflammatory players—macrophages, calcium, cholesterol, fibrous tissue—congregating on the scene of the blood vessel wall injury.

Lipoprotein

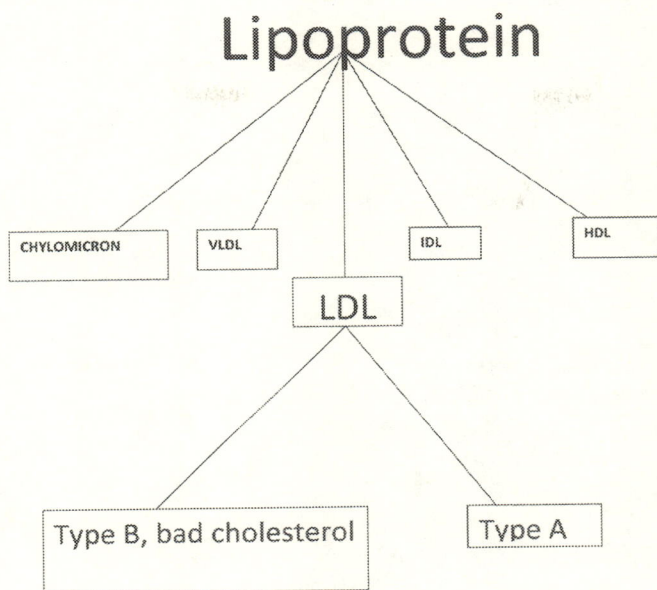

| CHYLOMICRON | VLDL | | IDL | | HDL |

LDL

Type B, bad cholesterol   Type A

Flow chart for types of lipoproteins

A vasculature scab, or plaque (also known as atheroma), develops as a result. The plaque creates more havoc, causing the affected arteries to rupture. Blood then leaks into the arterial walls and occludes its lumen (the cavity or channel within the arteries), depriving further blood flow to the heart muscles. A heart attack looms, and the pumping mechanism of the heart is in jeopardy of failing.

Obese individuals have greater risk for developing this condition because they are prone to producing fewer moieties that are protective and more moieties that are harmful to the inner walls of coronary arteries.

Chest pain is treated as an emergency—call 911—that requires prompt, aggressive evaluation and management.

CHAPTER 4

BMI and BMR

B ody mass index, or BMI, is a measurement of body fat as it relates to height and weight; that is, BMI helps to indicate if your weight is healthy for your height. Height must be taken into consideration before a conclusion is drawn as to whether a person is overweight. Two hundred pounds on a five-foot-five frame, for example, would be bursting at the seams, but that same weight on someone who is six foot five would look as flat as butter spread on a slice of bread. Estimating fat content in an individual became of paramount importance upon the realization that certain diseases are associated with overweight and obesity.

Many BMI calculators are available online—for instance, the National Institutes of Health offers this one: http://nhlbisupport.com/bmi/.

To find other calculators, just type "BMI" in an Internet search engine. When you know your BMI, determine whether your weight is normal by using the table below.

BMI	Category	comments
Less than 18.5	underweight	-------
18.5–24.9	normal	-------
25–29.9	overweight	increased health risk
30–34.9	obese	very high health risk
35 or higher	severe obesity	enormous health risk

You also can calculate your BMI based on the following equation:

Your weight in pounds
Your height inches^2 x 703

As an example, the following are my statistics before and after weight loss.

Before weight loss
Weight: 182 pounds
Height: 67 inches
Formula: weight in pounds divided by [height in inches]^2 multiplied by 703.
My BMI: 182 divided by $(67)^2$ x 703 = 28.5, which is overweight

After weight loss
Weight: 153 pounds
Height: 67 inches
My **current** BMI: 153 divided by $(67)^2$ x 703 = 23.8, which is normal.

Congratulations if your BMI is in the normal range. If it's high, you may have a runaway weight problem. Do not panic, but procrastinate no further. The purpose of this book is to show you how to approach the food you eat and the many options available to you in order to normalize your BMI.

BMR

Basal metabolic rate, or BMR, shows how our body spends the fuel energy in the food we eat. To be successful with weight loss, we need to understand all the components and dynamics that come together in this endeavor. We need to ask ourselves, how much food does a person really need? The concept of BMR will answer that question.

Food is the fuel that powers cellular and body functions. BMR is the energy our body needs to run its basic vital functions, such as heartbeat, digestion, kidney filtration, and mental effort. Obviously, the body needs fuel from food for things other than vital functions. It needs extra energy for additional activities, such as running, dancing, manual labor, bicycling, walking, typing, singing, and so forth. The amount of extra energy needed is commensurate with how physically exertional the activity is.

Knowing your BMR and daily calorie requirement provides a guide to how much food or calories your body needs to get through the day. If you eat more than your body needs, the excess food is stored in body as fat, and rapid weight gain occurs. For weight stability, a person's daily calorie intake (food and drink) must equal or approximate his or her daily calories burned (BMR, physical activities, and thermogenesis). Weight gain results if daily calorie intake is consistently greater than daily calories burned.

It turns out that the bulk of the calories we consume are for basal metabolic rate usage. The remainder of the daily calories ingested is applied to food digestion in the gut, muscular, and extraneous activities.

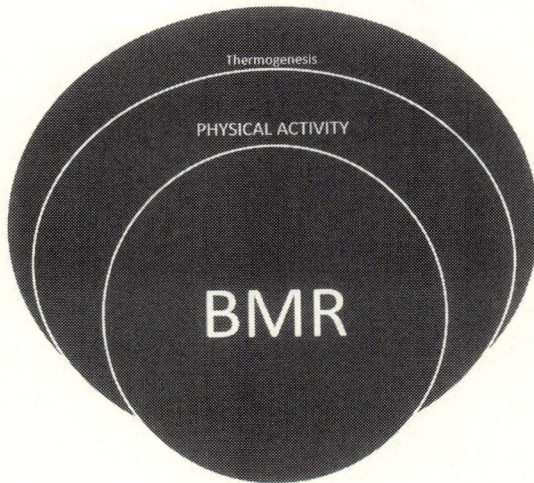

The above is an illustration of how daily calories are shared.

Suppose that you receive your daily calorie requirement at the beginning of the day. The illustration above shows the anticipated usage, with most of the calories applied to your BMR, with a quarter of them going for physical activities and only a tenth of the total daily calories committed to miscellaneous needs, also known as thermogenesis, which refers to grinding body heat generation that is not necessarily associated with vital organ functions. Food in excess of what the body needs is stored as fat and glycogen and contributes to the overall weight of the body. Food is needed mainly for BMR and physical activities.

BMR and daily calorie needs

The daily calorie need of an individual is determined by multiplying BMR with the person's activity factor. The following website offers an online calculator for determining daily calorie need: http://www.freedieting.com/tools/calorie_calculator.htm.

You also can calculate your daily calorie need using a mathematical formula. The formula for BMR is gender-specific. Other variables in the equation are age, height, and weight.

How to calculate individual BMR for men

66 + (6.23 x weight in pounds) + (12.7 x height in inches) − (6.8 x age in years)

How to calculate individual BMR for women

655 + (4.35 x weight in pounds) + (4.7 x height in inches) − (4.7 x age in years)

I will plug in my biometrics at age fifty to show how simple this formula is.

66 + (6.23 x 182 [weight in pounds]) + (12.7 x 67 [height in inches]) − (6 x 50 [age in years]) = **1750**

Calculate the daily calorie requirement

Once armed with your BMR, you are ready to estimate your daily calorie requirement by factoring in your activity level.

Level of activity	Activity factor	Comment
Sedentary	1.2	
Lightly active	1.375	
Moderately active	1.55	You exercise most days a week
Very active	1.725	You exercise intensely on a daily basis or for prolonged periods
Extremely active	1.9	You do hard labor or are in athletic training

As a physician, I consider my on-the-job and off-the-job activities as light; therefore, I multiply my BMR by a 1.375 factor to estimate my daily calorie need.

$$1750 \times 1.375 = 2406 \text{ calories}$$

Aging and BMR

Let us look at my BMR and daily caloric need as I aged from thirty years to sixty years, assuming all other factors are fairly stable.

Age	BMR	Calorie requirement
20	1855	2550
25	1881	2586
30	1870	2571
35	1813	2492
40	1810	2488
45	1745	2399

50	1750	2400
55	1677	2305
60	1643	2259

As mentioned above, I multiplied my BMR by 1.375 (light activity). Obviously, when calculating your daily calorie need for your weight, regardless of your age, you need to use the appropriate activity-level factor.

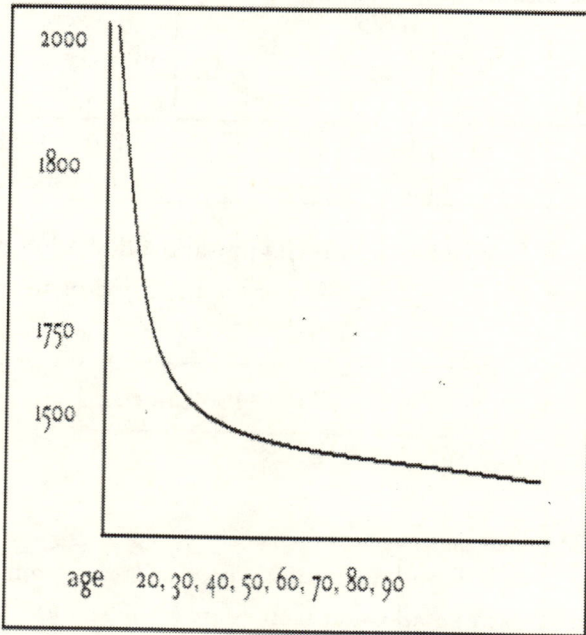

Graph of BMR and age

- X axis represents age; Y axis represents calories

The above graph, not drawn to scale, shows that between ages thirty and ninety, the BMR goes down very minimally. This means that caloric need will not vary much if activity level remains stable.

Interpreting the column

Notice that between age thirty and sixty, there is only a 312 [2571–2259] drop in the daily calorie need when activity level was constant at 1.375, but across the same age bracket of thirty to sixty, there is almost a 600-calorie drop [2571–1971] when activity level declined from light (1.375) to sedentary (1.2). This shows that activity level is very important, particularly as we age.

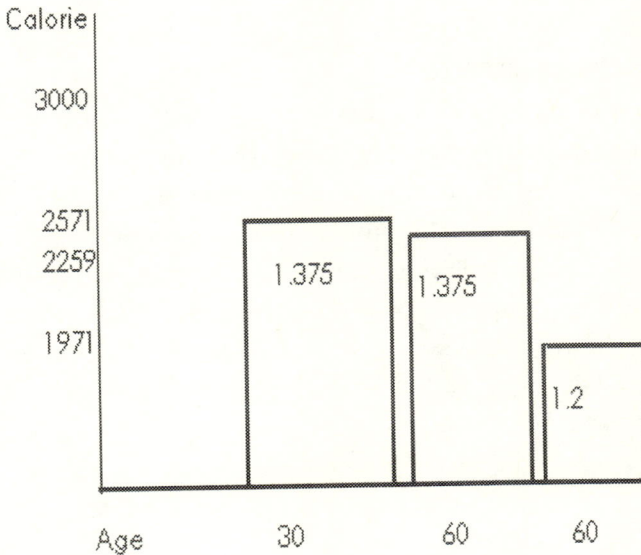

Relationship between calorie and activity level

The graph above shows the relationship between daily caloric need and activity level. Look at the near-normal level in daily calorie need at ages thirty and sixty. Compare that with a dramatic lowering of the calorie need when activity level drops from 1.375 to 1.2.

Blame activity level, not aging

As we age, our BMR slows down and our daily calorie requirement also drops. Age affects BMR in the loss of lean muscle mass, secondary to muscle atrophy. It is only logical that to maintain our weight when aging, we must decrease our calorie ingestion, reflective of our lowered BMR.

Activity level, more so than aging, has a greater impact on daily calorie requirement and weight gain. The surest way to rapid weight gain in the aging population is the "double whammy" of decreased activity and increased calories.

Higher BMR tends to correlate with burning calories and weight loss; conversely, lower BMR tends to correlate with increased calories and weight gain.

Weight loss and maintenance

Weight loss occurs if calorie intake is less than calorie expenditure. This negative calorie state enables the body to turn stored body fat into energy. Since stored fat contributes immensely to a person's weight, we tend to lose weight each time stored fat is used for energy.

To maintain lost weight, the calories in the food and beverages that you consume must approximate the calories you burn through BMR and physical activities. Any appreciable positive imbalance will tip the scale to weight gain.

CHAPTER 5

Do You Know What You Are Eating?

Food is to the body's cells as fuel is to an automobile. You wouldn't fill your car with bad gasoline, so why would you clog your cells with excessive and toxic food? Human cells produce the needed products and body parts, mend existing material, or destroy unwanted products. Because of the vital functions they serve in the body, cells need to function optimally, unimpeded by the influx of too much or toxic food.

Categories of food are not about the variety of food on the menu at your favorite restaurant. The composition of foods served by restaurants and fast-food outlets is different from the composition of food as it occurs in nature.

Standard food classification categorizes nature's food based on the main constituents, as in the table below.

Food Groups	Dominant Molecule	Comments
Grain	CHO, protein, fat	
Meat and protein	protein	
Dairy and related products	CHO, protein, fat	
Vegetable and fruits	CHO in fruit, protein in vegetables	
Fat and oil	fat	

Nuts	Fat, CHO, protein	
Water		Drink of choice
Beverages and drinks	Added sugar	Delete from menu
Junks, candies, and confectionaries	Added sugar	Delete from menu

General notes about food groups

- Each of the five major food groups is important. It is the quantity, the quality, and the frequency of eating these foods that contributes to excessive weight gain and obesity.
- There is no clear-cut rationale for putting a food type in a particular category. Food classification is based on source of origin, external appearance, and somewhat on the commonality of the predominant molecule: carbohydrate, protein, fat.
- Most food groups have a little bit of every molecule, but when a certain food item contains one predominant food molecule, it is usually put in that category. For example, an apple, classified under fruits, is mostly carbohydrates but also has some fat and plenty of minerals and vitamins. Peanut, a culinary nut in name only, is in the fat and oil category but also has a good amount of carbohydrates, protein, minerals, and vitamins. Meat has protein, but also fat, carbohydrates, and minerals.
- Choosing your food choice from different categories is essential in balancing the strengths and weakness of that particular food item.

My preference is to classify food as either natural or processed. This is a more useful food classification because the contrast is clear. Natural food is food in the form closest to its natural state, devoid of food processing. Processed food, on the other hand, means taking nature's own food and stripping it of much of its natural composition and/or contorting it into an unrecognizable form, with the intentions of making it more eye-catching to consumers and more lucrative to the food industries.

It turns out that every natural food group has its processed counterpart, a caricature built by the food industry. Some natural food has a genetically modified counterpart as well. *It is as if man thinks that he can do what nature has done.*

What does processing do to natural foods?

- destroys or disables food nutrients
- fills nature's food with habituating additives
- increases food calories

The questions to ask yourself are

- Would I trust nature's food as it is, or would I trust the food industry's remake of nature's food?
- Am I eating the natural form of my choice of food, or am I eating its processed form?

Dairy and dairy products

"Dairy," in this context, refers to milk, while "dairy products" refers to processed or refined foods derived from milk, such as ice cream, cheese, chocolate, and yogurt. Milk for human consumption comes mostly as cow milk and sometimes, especially in other cultures, from goats. The ease with which man has domesticated cows has made the use of cow's milk very popular and part of everyday nutrition.

Cow's milk contains mostly water. Its protein, fat, and carbohydrate contents are almost in equal proportion. The kind of fat contained in milk is the poor-quality saturated fat. The lactose in milk is glucose and galactose sugars combined. Milk also contains minerals and vitamins as detailed below:

- protein: 3.4 percent
- fat: 3.6 percent (mainly saturated fat, which is a poor-quality fat)
- sugar, lactose: 4.6 percent
- water: 87 percent
- minerals: calcium, magnesium, phosphorous, magnesium, potassium, sodium
- vitamins: fat-soluble—A, D, E, K; water-soluble—B, C, and folate (B vitamins include B1, thiamine; B2, riboflavin; B3, niacin; B5, pantothenic acid; B6, pyridoxine; and B12, cobalamine)

Like many other food groups, dairy products are often loaded with sugar or salt. Both salt and sugar are used for appetite appeal. Refined sugar in food stimulates appetite by causing upswings in the blood-sugar level. Sprinkling a few vitamins in processed dairy products is one trick employed by the food industries to bait consumers. Do not fall for that.

Lactose intolerance

People who suffer from lactose intolerance lack the ability to process the lactose sugar that is found in milk. When they drink milk or ingest milk products, such as ice cream or yogurt, they suffer from a bloated abdomen, loose stool, abdominal cramps, and nausea. Management includes avoiding milk and milk products and sometimes substituting cow's milk with lactose-free milk, such as soy milk or rice milk.

With cow's milk allergies, it is the protein component of the milk that triggers an immunological response. Signs and symptoms of cow's milk allergies are more systemic and may include nausea, vomiting, blood in the stool, eczema, wheezing, difficulty in breathing, and more. Management of this condition is more specialized and includes substituting cow's milk with nonmilk products and/or the use of highly digestible milk products. If you think you have an allergy to cow's milk, seek expert consultation.

Oil, fat, and related products

Oil occurs naturally in animal fat, plant seeds, and some plant leaves. Oil used for cooking is commonly extracted from both plant seeds and certain plant leaves. Animal fat is also a source of oil used in food preparation.

Oil, in most of its natural sources, has a combination of both saturated and unsaturated fat but in varying proportion. Plant sources of oil tend to have more of the unsaturated type of oil, while animal fat tends to have more of the saturated kind. Examples of plant sources of oil containing predominantly unsaturated fat include avocados, soybean, peanut, sunflower, olives, and cottonseeds.

In general, fat is used in baking to create moistness, cohesion, and to accentuate the taste of the other ingredients. Unsaturated fat is better for your health than saturated fat. Scientific literature shows saturated fat is detrimental to cardiovascular health, while unsaturated fat is thought to be somewhat protective to cardiovascular health. Though unsaturated fat is more wholesome than saturated fat, unsaturated fat is looked down upon by the food industry because it is not as stable and therefore is prone to faster decomposition and rancidity. Using saturated fat results in reduction in rancidity, which translates into increased shelf life and maximization of profits.

Animal fat and its products tend to contain lots of saturated fat and should be avoided. Like animal fat, certain plant foods also contain high amounts of saturated fat and as such carry some cautionary notes in their consumption. These include coconut oil, chocolate, palm kernel oil, and cottonseed oil.

Olive fruits and flaxseed are prototypes of plant sources of oil. Both contain more unsaturated fat than saturated fat. The unsaturated fat in olives includes mono- and polyunsaturated fat: omega-3 and omega-6 fatty acids and variable amounts of vitamins, especially E and K. Flaxseed contains unsaturated fat, including linolenic acid, oleic acid, omega-3, omega-6, and omega-9. The omega fatty acids are interesting because they are purported to have some cardio-protective, inflammatory, and immune modulation properties.

Hydrogenation is the process often employed by food industries to turn unsaturated oil and fat into saturated oil and fat. Turning unsaturated fat, such as vegetable oil (nature's own oil) to saturated fat (the food industry's choice) by bombarding it with hydrogen (hydrogenation) introduces undesirable trans fat. Trans fat has been cited as contributing to diseases ranging from coronary artery disease to some forms of cancers.

Meat and protein

The meat on your dinner plate comes from a variety of mammals—cattle, lamb, goat, pig, chicken, turkey. Individual preferences often depend on the type of meat someone was introduced to as a child or what is available or affordable at any given moment. Some cultures eat dog, snails, snake, rabbit, and deer. Famine and poverty sometimes can expand the list of mammals that are consumed. Generally speaking, meats contain 19 percent protein and 75 percent water. Meat also contains other food macromolecules and ingredients such as fat, 3 percent carbohydrates, and 1 percent minerals and vitamins. Unlike plant foods, meat has more saturated fat than unsaturated fat.

Composition of goat meat

- protein: 19 percent
- fat: 3 percent
- carbohydrate: 1 percent
- minerals: 2 percent: zinc, iron, selenium, and phosphorous
- vitamins: B12, B6, niacin, choline, and riboflavin
- water: 75 percent

Opponents of animal protein consumption recognize that protein is important for the body but advocate that it should be consumed from plant sources rather than animal sources. They blame animal protein as the root cause of many health maladies, ranging from cancer to autoimmune diseases. Some people dislike eating animals due to the humane reason that mammals are closely related to humans in terms of evolutionary hierarchy and intelligence. They argue that even the wildest mammals can be domesticated as pets and companions. Other reasons for not eating meat include the following:

- There is an increasing realization that plant protein is superior, healthier, and better suited for human well-being than animal protein.
- Sodium nitrite used in meat coloring and preservation can degenerate to nitrosamine when heated. And nitrosamine has been thought to be carcinogenic.
- Unwholesome meat products can come from multiple sources, such as chicken nuggets, where tiny pieces of chicken are thickly coated with salt and fried oil.

Mad cow disease

Mad cow disease is an animal disease that can be transmitted to humans. In this disease, a naturally occurring protein in the cow, called prion, goes berserk and folds abnormally. As a result of this protein malfunction, the cows become neurologically sick, with symptoms such as aggression, irritability, and apathy. More cows become affected when they are fed meats and bones from affected cows.

Signs may not show up in affected cows for years. Humans who eat the affected meat become ill. Some of the signs and symptoms of mad cow disease in humans include memory loss, malaise, fatigue, numbness, muscle spasms, difficulty in concentration, depression, and hallucinations.

Grains and legumes

If you come across a small but hard seed in a whole-food store, the chances are that you are looking at a grain. Grains and legumes are similar in nutrient content. Grains are seeds of grasses, while legumes are seeds from the bean family. Unlike grains, which are one whole unit, legumes tend to have a tendency to split externally through their coat or internally along their seeds.

Grain is arguably the most balanced of all the stand-alone food groups. If you want to choose a single food group to take on a trip, grain should be the top choice. Whole grains contain adequate amounts of carbohydrates, protein, fibers, and some fat. In addition, they contain lots of vitamins and minerals.

In its entirely natural form, whole grains are made up of germ, endosperm, and bran. Most of the minerals and vitamins are contained in the bran and the germ. During food processing, lots of these vital nutrients are lost. Attempts to shore up the quality of processed grain by adding lost nutrients often fall very short.

Oat, soybean, corn, wheat, barley, millet, rye, and mustard are examples of grains. Choose from grains—powerful nature's food—next time you plan your meal. Beans, lentils, peanuts are good examples of legumes. Soybeans are legumes with a high fat content.

Oat, as the prototype of a grain, contains:

- protein: variable from 10–40 percent
- carbohydrate: 30–70 percent of starch and sugar
- fat: 2–5 percent
- fibers: 3–12 percent
- minerals: magnesium, iron, zinc, potassium, calcium, iron, sodium, manganese, copper
- vitamins: B vitamins (niacin, folic acid, panthothenic acid, thiamine) and vitamins K and E

As mentioned, food processing shreds the component parts of grain, destroying its essential nutrients. You can notice these processed grains packaged in colorful boxes as cereals, enclosed in shiny wrappers as whole wheat breads, camouflaged in deceptive advertisements as authentic, and positioned on store shelves as ready-to-eat. But they are loaded with refined sugar and sprinkled with synthetic vitamins.

Due to the high-fiber content of natural grains, among other healthful qualities, consumption of whole, natural grains is recommended by many nutritionists.

Fruits and vegetables

Fruits can be defined as the edible part of a plant that harbors its seed. A basketful of assorted fruits would display a panoply of color, size, taste, shape, texture, aroma, and beauty. Fruits range in texture from the softies, such as tomatoes and oranges, to those that are dry, such as coconuts. While some fruits, such as apples and pears, grow as a single fruit, others, such as grapes and bananas, grow in bunches. There are giant-looking fruits, such as watermelon, squash, pumpkin, cantaloupe, and pineapple. Explore the world of fruits.

Vegetables are easily recognized as the edible part of a plant. But not everybody notices the many other food groups that are under this category. Indeed any edible part of a plant, with the exclusion of its fruits and nuts, can be classified as a vegetable. This umbrella will accommodate plant-derived foods such as potatoes, sprouts, stems, carrots, beets, onions, asparagus, and yams. It is essential to appreciate this, as most of these plant-derived foods are nutritious and satisfying.

Herbs

Herbs can be described as vegetables with a sharp aroma. As such, they are added in meals as seasoning for flavor and taste. One person's vegetable could be another person's herbs. Thyme, parsley, and basil are example of herbs. Others include the leaves of oregano, linden, eucalyptus, and peppermint. The oil of thyme, an essential plant oil, has some medicinal properties. Herbs are perhaps best suited to indigenous experience, which in some instances span thousands of years across many generations.

Health

Both fruits and leafy vegetables contain similar nutrients, as both are derivatives of the plant. Both contain the good, complex carbohydrates, as well as fiber, proteins, vitamins, minerals, and phytochemicals. *They contain very little fat.* Carbohydrates occur more in fruits than in vegetables. Quantity and quality of nutrients in fruits and vegetables tend to vary across different climatology and geography.

Phytochemicals

Phytochemicals are groups of biochemically active substances of unquantifiable efficacy that are responsible for some of the colors and scents found in fruits and vegetables. Lycopene is a well-known phytochemical found in tomatoes and is thought to have a positive effect on prostate health.

Spinach is a prototype of vegetables. Spinach contains lots of vitamins, minerals, fiber, some carbohydrates, and some fat, as well as omega-3 and omega-6 fatty acids.

Edible derivatives of plant root

The capability of plants to store food in parts of their stems and roots is enormous. At many levels beneath the soil, new roots sprout and diverge from the main root. Some of these roots will store the food the plants need during an austere period. These are known as storage, or tuberous, roots. Those endowed with large storage capacity, like yams, serve as main meals, while those with lean storage capacity, like gingerroot, serve as spices.

Man takes advantage of plant food when he harvests them and cooks them so that they are edible. The list of plants' derived food is long and are known by different names in different parts of the world. Their nutritious qualities are comparable to each other. They contain water, complex carbohydrates, and a variable amount of fiber, protein, vitamins, and minerals.

Many plants have been found to have bioactive ingredients that can affect human health. Some are used solely for their medicinal properties.

Highly specialized plant stems, like turmeric, which is one of the main ingredients in curry, contain essential plant oil. Horseradish roots have culturally recognizable curative and medicinal properties.

Tuberous root derivatives include yam, cassava or yucca, mauka, and potato.

Tap-root derivatives are carrots, celeriac, beets, and radishes.

Plant-bulb derivatives, such as onions and garlic, are used as spices in meals.

Plant-stem derivatives include sugarcane, ginseng, and turmeric.

Cocoyam and eddoe (also known as malanga) are derivatives of the plant corm—the stout, underground part of the plant stem used for food storage.

Personal note

In the village of Akokwa, Nigeria, where I grew up, we used *mpoto ede,* the broad leaf of cocoyam, as an umbrella. The liquid of the cocoyam leaves, however, can cause severe itching. It was a child's greatest nightmare to be contaminated with the itchy fluid from the cocoyam leaves. Its itch is comparable to a severe case of poison ivy.

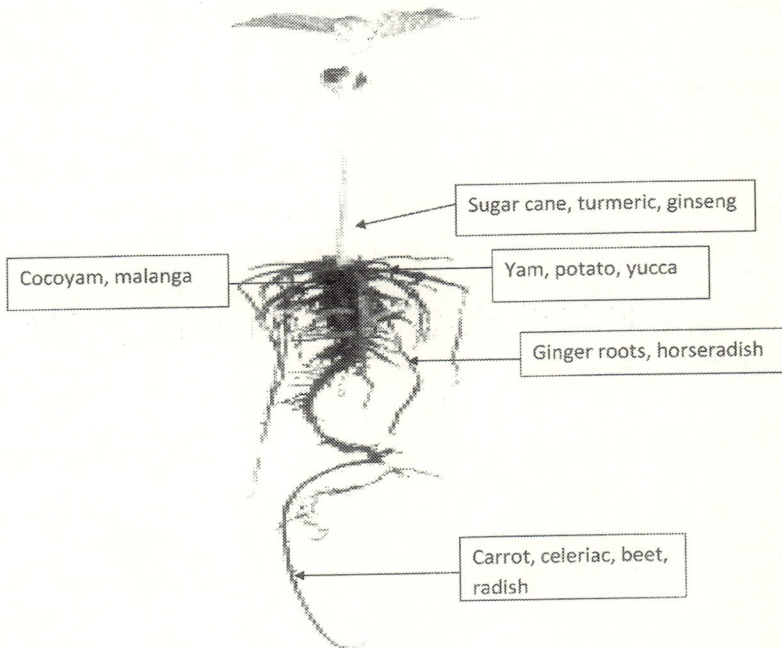

Graph showing some derivatives of plant food

Nuts

Scouting for nuts in the store and trying to identify them correctly was an exciting part of my research in writing this book. Nuts nomenclature is confusing, because there are true nuts, in a botanical sense, and there are culinary nuts, in a food sense. Don't let that drive you nuts. Sometimes, it is not clear how to classify a nut; for example, coconut can be classified as a fruit, a nut, or a seed. Irrespective of the classification, it is sufficient to know that nuts contain mainly fat, minerals, protein, sugar, and fiber.

Some nuts—the true nuts—have both a hard coat and inseparable seeds, while others, the culinary nuts, may have soft coats and separable seeds. One of the common characteristics of nuts is that they are hard to crack. Many of the local food stores I visited were selling walnuts, almonds, hazelnuts and chestnuts.

Most of the fuss about nuts has to do with nut allergies. Although peanuts are technically legumes, most people think of them as nuts. A peanut allergy is common and can be life-threatening. It's important to recognize the signs and symptoms of a nut allergy. Symptoms can range from mild irritation of the throat to a body rash to lip and facial swelling and shortness of breath. Individuals who experience symptoms of a nut allergy should seek immediate medical attention. It's recommended that people who have nut allergies should carry an EpiPen (epinephrine) at all times in case of anaphylaxis, a severe allergic reaction that threatens breathing.

Below is a table comparing nutritional values of vegetable, fruits, and nuts.

	Vegetables, leafy	Fruits	Nuts
Minerals	especially iron, calcium		
Vitamins	K	especially C	
Antioxidants			
Phytochemical			
Fiber	insoluble, soluble	soluble	insoluble

Sugar, Carbohydrate	variable		
Fats	minimal	minimal, *with the exception of avocado and olives*	unsaturated
Protein	variable		

Summary

- Naturally occurring carbohydrates can be found mostly in grains, in legumes, in dairy, in fruits and vegetables, in nuts, and somewhat in meat.
- Naturally occurring protein can be found, in order of abundance, in grains and legumes, in meat, in milk, in vegetables and fruits,
- Naturally occurring fat, oil, or lipids occur abundantly in some plants and plant seeds and animal fat.
- Vegetables, fruits, grains, legumes, nuts, and, to some extent, milk have an abundance of minerals, vitamins, antioxidants, and phytochemicals.
- Leafy vegetables and most fruits, with some notable exceptions (avocados, coconuts, and olives), have minimal to no fat content.
- Of all the naturally occurring food groups, nuts contain the most amount per gram of fat, but fats found in nuts are proportionately higher in the favored unsaturated fat, rather than saturated fat. Animal fat contains mostly saturated fat.

CHAPTER 6

Sugar, Salt, and Food Labels

Refined sugar often is added to the food we eat. Added sugar is in breads, jams, canned foods, cereals, chocolate bars, candies, and so forth. Today's shelved foods are little more than clumps of decorated sugar. Soft drinks are essentially liquid sugar. Refined sugar is derived from sugarcane, which is a giant grass that grows in the tropics. I ate a lot of sugarcane when I was a kid growing up in Nigeria. Sugarcane contains sucrose, but before sucrose can become table sugar, it undergoes a series of refining processes.

A certain level of sugar in the blood is acceptable and normal. *Glycemia* refers to the presence of an excess level of sugar (glucose) in the blood. Certain foods, especially those with lots of added sugar, can cause a sudden upswing in the blood sugar level. Such foods are said to have a high glycemic index. These are distinguished from foods with a low glycemic level index—complex carbohydrates—that lead to a gradual increase rather than a sudden upswing in the blood sugar level.

The problem with a sudden upswing in the blood sugar level is that it triggers a sudden release of the hormone insulin to deal with all that sugar. The rapid release of insulin causes a sudden drop in blood sugar level, which creates a sensation of hunger, making one more likely to consume more of the sugar-sweetened food. The cycle is repeated over and over again if you continue to flood your body with high glycemic meals.

The hormone insulin is produced by the pancreas. The constant demand for the pancreas to churn out insulin to deal with all that refined sugar flooding the blood may eventually cause the pancreas to fail. When the pancreas fails, insulin production is compromised. Blood sugar cannot be handled adequately. At this stage, a person will likely develop type 2 diabetes. Without adequate medical intervention, type 2 diabetes causes a constant elevation of blood sugar in the body. Diabetes is a systemic illness with ramifications that are felt in the entire body. Eating foods with a low glycemic can prevent or delay the onset of type 2 diabetes.

Why is there so much sugar in refined food? The answer to this question may lie within capitalism—money and profits transcend any other consideration, regardless of health consequences. If sugar sells food, manufacturers will pour in as much sugar as they can in the food they sell. The goal is to tantalize the consumers with sugar, to draw out their taste buds, and create the desire for more sugary products. The food industry is polluting the cellular functions within us.

On October 23, 2012, Michael Pollan said in a radio interview on WBAI's *Democracy Now!* program that every new onset of type 2 diabetes could cost New York City four hundred thousand dollars. He blamed excessive consumption of soda as one of the major contributing factors to the rising incidence of type 2 diabetes. He supported New York mayor Michael Bloomberg's effort to limit the quantity of soda consumed as part of the fight to combat this epidemic.

Added sugar is empty calories, because it has no nutrient value. Compare added sugar in processed foods with the natural sugar content in fruits, which also provide vitamins, minerals, and antioxidants. It is prudent to avoid refined sugar of all kinds at all times.

How many empty calories are you getting from added sugar? Bear in mind that:

- 1 tsp. of sugar equals 4 grams
- 1 gram of sugar equals 3.87 calories
- 1 tsp. of sugar equals 3.87 x 4 = 15.48 calories

Let's apply this to a chocolate bar. Take a store-brand chocolate bar. There are six servings per bar; the sugar content per serving is 24 grams. This means that if you ate all the chocolate, you would be consuming 144 grams of sugar, which is equivalent to 36 teaspoons of sugar, because one teaspoon of sugar equals 4 grams—and 144 grams of sugar has 557 calories.

Let's take bread as another example. A serving size is two slices, with 4 grams of sugar in each serving. Look at the table below as you track the number of slices you eat with the grams of sugar—and the calories—you consume.

Number of slices eaten	Grams of sugar eaten	*Calories in sugar alone*
2	4	15.48
4	8	30.96
8	16	61.92
12	*24, six tsp	92.88
16	32	123.8
18	**36, nine tsp	139.3

* Daily limit of added sugar for men, as recommended by the American Heart Association
** Daily limit of added sugar for women, as recommended by the American Heart Association

By eating twelve slices of bread—equivalent to six teaspoons of sugar—you will have reached your daily recommended sugar limit for the day. I have no doubt that the food industry is competing for who will add the most sugar for sale. No wonder the kids are overweight and society is facing a diabetic epidemic.

Do not worry about depleting the sugar in your body if you stop ingesting refined sugar. Fruits, vegetables, grains, and tubers are some of the natural sources of sugar.

Salt

Table salt—sodium chloride—is made up of the elements sodium and chlorine. Both elements, especially sodium, are vital in human body physiology, where they play a role in cell membrane transportation, cell-to-cell communication, impulse propagation, and other effects. Sodium is also vital in the maintenance of the fluid equilibrium in the body's intravascular and extravascular fluid spaces.

Most of the salt on the dinner table is from the sea. To make it to the store shelves for sale, the sea-dredged salt has to undergo a refining process, which includes washing and bleaching. Table salt is available as iodized (containing iodine) or as noniodized. Using iodized table salt is a convenient way to give our bodies the element iodine, an essential trace element used by the thyroid gland to produce the hormones thyroxin and triiodothyronine. The absence of iodine in the diet and failure of the thyroid gland to produce the needed thyroid hormones may lead to a low-functioning thyroid gland and to the enlargement of the thyroid gland, known as a goiter. Some of the symptoms of a low-functioning thyroid gland, or hypothyroidism, may include fatigue, depression, cold intolerance, or mental retardation in children. Using iodized salt has been a successful way to combat this problem.

The food industry has usurped the essence of table salt as a way to provide iodine in the diet; it uses salt to control consumer taste and consumer appetite for purchasing and devouring more of the salt-loaded food. Salt is also used as a preservative to extend food shelf life and to prevent or mask rapid food decay.

There are health consequences to excess salt in food. Too much sodium can shift the delicate fluid system in our body's physiology toward expansion of the intravascular fluid. Chronic fluid shift and retention could lead to high blood pressure and other ills associated with hypertension—for example, stroke.

Half a teaspoon of iodized salt, containing about 190 mcg of iodine, is all that is needed to meet the body's daily iodine requirement. Younger people may need a little bit less, while pregnant and breast-feeding women may need a little more. Tracking how much sodium and salt you eat is difficult, because lots of commonly available food—pizza, hot dogs, soups, hamburgers, fries, bread, chips—are deliberately sprayed with salt for sensation inducement. Sprinkling a large order of fries with one teaspoon of salt is almost all the salt a person needs for the day.

Paying attention to food labels or preparing your own food is a good way of estimating and monitoring how much sodium you ingest.

Natural sources of sodium include seafood, fish, and meat. Celery is an example of a vegetable that contains lots of sodium. Natural sources of iodine include seafood, clams, oysters, turnips, shrimp, cod, saltwater fish, and sea vegetable (e.g., kelp). Milk and egg yolks also contain iodine.

Recommendations

- Make a conscious effort to diversify your food categories.
- Be aware of what you are eating. Take notice of the content of your meal.
- Do not assume that the restaurateur gives a damn about your health. The chances are that he cares more about his finances than your well-being. Make specific demands when you eat at a restaurant. Ask for no salt and no sugar. Ask for low-fat or fat-free milk.
- Be diversified in your daily meals.
- Include fruits, vegetables, and grains in your daily menu. They contain lots of vitamins and phytochemicals that may help augment your immune system. It worked for me. Even the flu virus could not touch me this year.

Food labels

View food labels as a marketing medium through which the food sellers appeal to patrons. Labels may contain some element of the truth, but they are largely tilted toward deception and exaggeration.

Just because a food label uses the words "slim" or "healthy" does not mean that the food vendors have any interest in your health. Have your eyes wide open when reading food labels. Never forget that food sellers are only interested in making some bucks off you. Look at all the components of the food on the label—fat and sugar but also fiber, vitamins, salt, additives, preservatives, and so forth.

Interpreting the label's fat content

Evaluate not only the total calories from fat but also the type of fat in the food—saturated or unsaturated. If an item's food label contains a high percentage of saturated fat, stay away from it. It is a signal that this particular food manufacturer does not care much about nutritional health. Take, for example, peanut butter "for dieters": the label indicates a two-tablespoon serving size contains 32 grams of fat. How many calories do you think two tablespoons of "peanut butter for dieters" spread on your sandwich will add to your body system? To start, note that 1 gram of fat generates 9 calories. Therefore, two tablespoons of this peanut butter, containing 32 grams of fat, yields 288 calories.

Fat recap

Saturated fat is mainly a derivative of animal fat or a product of hydrogenation from plant-based oil. It is mostly unhealthy. You will recollect from previous chapters that the food industry uses saturated fat to reduce food decay and prolong shelf life. However, saturated fat obtained by hydrogenation contains trans fat, which is harmful to cardiovascular health.

Even though 1 gram of fat gives 9 calories of energy when eaten, it takes fewer calories, about 7.7 calories of exertion, to get rid of 1 gram of fat from the body. This is because stored body fat is not all fatty; it is mired with tissue water, protein, and fiber, making it a tad less arduous to burn.

So if it takes 7.7 calories of effort to dislodge 1 gram of fat in your body, how many calories does it take to burn a pound of fat?

Note that one pound is equal to 454 grams. Since one pound of body weight is equivalent to 454 grams, it will take approximately 3,495 calories' (7.7 x 454) worth of exertion to get rid of one pound of fat weight in the body.

Recommended

Item	Daily Recommendation	Equivalence/Comment
salt	not more than 6 grams (1 tsp.) of salt	Only 1 tsp. of table salt, or 6 grams of salt
sugar	not more than 100–150 calories	not more than 9 tsp. per day, or 37.5 gram/day
soda	treat as sugar	12 ounces of regular soda contains 8 tsp. of sugar and is about 130 calories
fiber	20–38 grams	in grains and vegetable
fruits	2–3 cups	easy on it
vegetables	2–3 cups	eat liberally
vitamin	strongly consider daily vitamins	especially if you are not food diversified
saturated fat	less than 7% of total calories	use as litmus test
trans fat	less than 1% of total calories	
water	1–3 liters	4–12 cups, variable

CHAPTER 7

Weight Dynamics and Macronutrients

The human body is made up of:
1. Water: 65 percent
2. Protein: 15 percent
3. Fat: 15 percent
4. Miscellaneous: 5 percent (mostly minerals such as calcium, potassium, sodium)
5. Carbohydrate: less than 1 kg

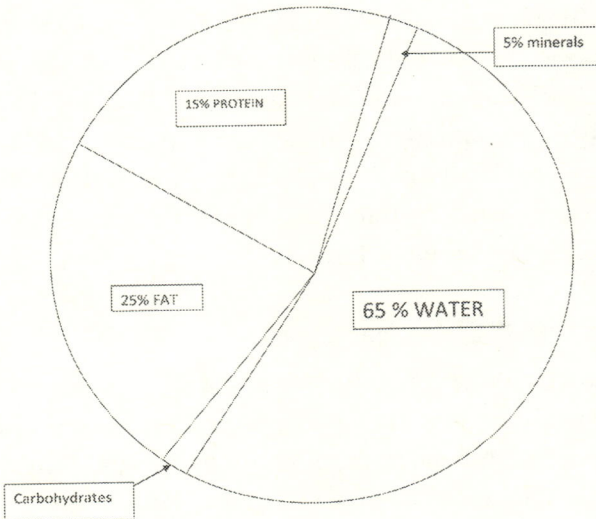

Pie diagram of human body weight distribution

The pie chart shows how a person's total weight is broken down (not drawn to scale). Notice that most of what is in a person's weight is water, followed by fat and protein in almost equal proportion, and then minerals. Carbohydrate is responsible for a negligible portion of a human weight. This is because the body would rather channel its supply of carbohydrate as fuel.

As previously mentioned, weight gain occurs when calorie intake exceeds calorie expenditure. Food calories in excess of what the body needs are converted to fat and stored in the adipose tissue. Fat is the most efficient way the body stores excess calories. Weight fluctuation, whether it is a gain or a loss, occurs from this pool of shifting fat stores in the body.

Water accounts for up to 60 percent of a person's weight. Most of the body's water is equally divided between the intracellular space and extracellular spaces. Intracellular water is the water inside the cells, while extracellular water is water in the blood vessels, joints, intestinal spaces, and body cavities. The mechanism of thirst, water intake, and water excretions through urination ensures that body water is in a fair balance. Body water remains in equilibrium unless in extreme conditions, such as entrapment and disease conditions when the body compensates and water loss occurs in both spaces.

Fluctuation in a person's weight is almost exclusively due to the fat component. If someone's weight increases, it is most likely that person has added tremendously to the proportion of fat in his or her body. This is because calories in excess of what the body needs are converted to fat. For this reason, although almonds are a healthy snack, do not eat a massive amount of almonds and expect to lose weight. That will be impossible. Excess carbohydrate ingestion, greater than what the body needs, is quickly converted to fat.

Macronutrients and their recommendation

Macronutrients refer to fat, protein, and carbohydrate in our food. Below is the recommendation for major food groups for ages nineteen and older. The recommendation for children is slightly different: 5–20 percent less protein and 30–40 percent more fat.

Complex carbohydrates are recommended the most because this is the fuel most efficient for providing our body with needed daily energy for activities and BMR.

Dietary recommendation of major macronutrients:
- carbohydrates, 45–65 percent
- fat, 20–35 percent
- protein, 10–35 percent

In every food group, all the macronutrients are important. Some of the fundamental benefits in each of the major food macronutrients are listed below.

Functions of fat
Fat serves various functions in the body, including the following:
1. Under the skin, fat serves as insulation against cold and hypothermia.
2. In a measured amount, fat serves as a beauty mold to facial features. (Imagine the unattractive gaunt look of a fat-free face.)
3. Fat serves as a source of energy for the body.
4. Fat serves as a vital vehicle in the absorption of fat-soluble vitamins.
5. Fat is a vital component of cellular structure and cellular messengers.

Table showing fat-soluble vitamins

Vitamin	Chemical name	Deficiency disease
Vitamin A	retinol	night blindness
Vitamin D	cholecalciferol	rickets and scurvy
Vitamin E	tocopherol	anemia
Vitamin K	phylloquinone	hemorrhage

These vitamins can only be absorbed in the body in the presence of fat.

Essential fatty acids

Fatty acids (some of which are shown below) are essential to the body, which implies that these groups of fatty acids must be part of the normal diet, as the body cannot make them.

Omega-3 fatty acid— alphalinolenic acid	Found mostly in seeds and vegetable oil; has cardio-protective effects; inflammatory and immune modulation capacity
Omega-6 fatty acid—linolenic acid	Found in vegetable oil; has inflammatory and immune-modulation properties
Gamma-linolenic acid	From seeds and vegetable oil; somewhat essential. Also has some inflammatory and immune-modulation characteristics.
Lauric acid	Somewhat essential. Found in coconut oil, palm kernel oil, and breast milk. May increase the good cholesterol.
Palmetoleic acid, omega-7	Found in animal, vegetable, and marine oil. High amounts in the liver. Somewhat essential; may play a role in obesity.

Functions of carbohydrates

Carbohydrates provide efficient energy fuel to the body (1 gram of sugar carbohydrate yields 4 calories of energy).

Carbohydrates are also part of cell genetic facet in the form of ribose sugar, present as deoxyribose nucleic acid of DNA.

In the forms of oligosaccharides, a few monosaccharides linked together, carbohydrates act as cell recognition tags for cell-to-cell interaction, signaling, and communication.

Functions of protein

Muscle tissue is a good example of a body structure that is made up predominantly of protein. But as shown in the table below, protein is widely integrated in human functionality and structure.

Functions of proteins	Location and comment
As a depot	Casein in cow and human milk stores calcium and phosphorous; ferritin stores iron
As protection for body invaders	Complements and provides antibodies for the immune system
Mobility	Actin and myosin in muscles
Signal and communication	Hormones such as insulin and glucagon
Identification	Human leukocyte antigen for tissue recognition
Metabolism	Catalysts and enzymes in human physiology
Transport proteins	Cytochromes transfer electrons during tissue respiration; hemoglobin transports oxygen
Provides support for body structures	In nails, skin, and hair

The ten essential amino acids

Amino acids are the building blocks of protein, so their functions fit into the general functions of proteins. However, some of the amino acids—the essential amino acids—deserve to be highlighted.

There are twenty different types of amino acids to choose from in the building of all the structural and morphological types of protein that occur in nature. Only ten of the twenty known amino acids are thought to be essential, in that the body cannot make them, and therefore they must be ingested through food. The other ten are nonessential because the body can make them. Since amino acids are protein, all of the ten can be gotten from protein-containing foods, such as eggs, fish, legumes, nuts, seeds, beef, and milk.

The table below shows the essential ten.

Essential amino acids	Food source	Notable function	Comments
phenylalanine	egg, fish, legumes, nuts, seeds, beef, milk	precursor for dopamine, norepinephrine, and epinephrine synthesis	dopamine and epinephrine are important neurotransmitters in the body
valine	same		
threonine	same		
tryptophan	same	elaborates serotonin and vitamin B3	increase in serotonin helps combat insomnia, depression, and anxiety
isoleucine	same	general protein function (GPF)	
methionine	same	GPF	
histidine	same	help heal wounds	
arginine	same	GPF	
leucine	same	GPF	
lysine	same	GPF	

CHAPTER 8

Confronting the Weight Challenge

Our body is in decay-default mode—this means that, biologically speaking, our body is preset to gain weight as we get older, become soggy, and die. Deliberate actions must be taken to delay or control some of these natural body tendencies.

The body resembles a mechanical motor, tiring and wearing out as we age, for which extra care and efficiency has to be employed to prolong life span. Giving the body the right food in the right amount will go a long way to improving our quality of life.

Weight management should take a holistic dimension that starts with recognition and a set of action plans and strategies to combat and confront it. The main target is food—both the quantity and quality. The second target is physical activities, both frequency and intensity.

Do not sweep an increased-weight issue under the carpet. It is too big a health risk not to tackle it. Many people realize how overweight they are and talk about doing something about it or even going the extra mile of taking action, but unfortunately, many still quickly fall by the wayside. To prevent giving up quickly, one needs to understand why it is necessary to embark on this journey and understand the challenges ahead.

Listen to your body

Part of listening to your body is to avoid food types that cause you to gain weight. You are the first to notice how you feel, but you must learn how to listen to your body. Medical practitioners do not know what you are feeling if you do not let them know. This is the reason why clinicians begin consultations by eliciting information from patients. Insights garnered from self-observation are very valuable; for instance, many people who avoid certain foods instinctively have been proven to be allergic to them.

Take an inventory

Take an inventory of your food habits. Write out a list of what goes into your body each day, and be as thorough and systematic as you can. Capture as many food bad habits as you can. It may take you a couple of days or so, and if some forgotten bad food habit pops up in your brain in the future, write it down. Such an inventory is a benchmark of where you are at the moment so you can compare it with what changes and accomplishments you will make in the future. Below is a sample of my own catharsis:

1. I forgot the relationship between health and weight.
2. I constantly indulged in fast food and refined food.
3. I never paid attention to what was in the food I ate.
4. I was too busy to prepare my own food.
5. I let my body dictate what I ate.
6. I fed myself unhealthy food at home.
7. I made bad choices in what I ate and in what I drank.
8. I had no time for exercise
9. Snacks accompanied me on every trip I made.
10. I had an insatiable, uncontrollable appetite.

A good food-habit inventory will reveal how you got into your weight predicament. Have fun with it—tease yourself and have a belly laugh about how ignorant you were. You must follow up with a resolution to make significant changes and be committed to stay on track.

Tackle the obvious first

Nutritional habits such as drinking soft drinks or eating boxes of refined cereal and buckets of fried foods are outright bad. Cut them off immediately. Your body will quickly regulate to that lifestyle change. I had my own indulgence. Oil-fried plantain was my delicacy of choice. I prepared it and ate it for years. I watched the weight stick on me, year in, year out. Eventually, I had to let that go. It has been over one year since I ate fried plantain. Surprisingly, I do not miss it. I occasionally eat plantain, but it has to be boiled or baked.

Replace old bad habits with new good habits

Trimming your weight to within normal limits and maintaining it should neither be very mystifying nor an impossible task. First, identity all your bad eating habits and indulgences, and second, replace them with healthier choices.

Many of us may be fooled by what we consider healthy foods; even science sometimes gets it wrong. But there are many foods and food habits that have been validated as deleterious to health, and it behooves us to shun them or at least limit their consumption. Cigarettes, alcohol, refined sugar, junk food, salty food, candies, processed food, soda, and refined cereals are some notable examples.

Dress up your food in a manner that is attractive. My daughter will eat a cut-up apple but will shy away from one whole, big apple—both the same apple, but each presenting different visuals.

I am not a nitpicker for portioning and rationing, as long as one eats naturally occurring nonprocessed food. Go ahead; have as many vegetables as you can. Go ahead and have as moderate an amount of fruit as your stomach will allow. Go ahead and enjoy your cooked beans and brown rice until you are full. Even as I challenge you to enjoy your naturally occurring food to your fullest, I will point out that too much of a good thing is bad, so eat in moderation. Avoid stretching your stomach to bloated capacity. Be ready to finish eating at the earliest signal that you are full. Take cues from your stomach. You probably have eaten too much if, in the course of a normal meal, you feel the urge to throw up. I do not particularly like the aspect of a plate size as a way of gauging what we eat. We are already equipped with a stomach, a sophisticated gauge wired to the brain. If we do not adhere to what our stomach is telling us, I doubt whether the plate can do any better controlling our desire for food.

"Broccoli-Head" and food rotation

Before I changed my bad food habits I knew about broccoli and that it is touted as the super vegetable, packed with antioxidants, vitamins, and minerals. I bought into it and ate lots of broccoli every day for weeks and months. It so happened that on one happy night, my wife smelled my head and screamed out, "Broccoli-Head!" I laughed for a good minute. That got me to appreciate the importance of food rotation. Endeavor to diversify your choices even within each food group.

Food rotation not only provides impetus and variety, but it also fulfills the subtle nutritional differences between food groups and even within individual groups and types. Be creative. It is fun to go from apples to peas, to peaches, to oranges, to avocados. Food rotation also guards against the tendency to be hooked on a particular food item. Make your cellular machineries versatile by eating a variety of natural food.

JADE it: Jettison Appetizer and DEssert

A couple of years ago, I stopped partaking in appetizers and desserts. When my companions munch away on a basket of bread and butter, I enjoy sips of cold water, sometimes with a slice of lemon. With the expanding size of main dishes, nobody truly needs an appetizer or a dessert. Most people come to the dinner table because they are hungry. An appetizer is not going to whip up any more appetite than already exists, but it will surely add to your caloric intake and weight gain. The same goes with dessert.

Count your calories

It's important to know your daily caloric need so that you can determine whether you are meeting or exceeding it. Approximate calorie content of many recipes is available in some restaurants. This information can be found in an Internet search. Try to tally your daily calories. After a while, you will know the calorie range of what you eat. View that against your calorie requirement for age and activity. Make the necessary adjustment to get within your caloric range.

Fasting

Fasting won't harm you unless you have a medical condition or you are taking certain medications that preclude fasting. Fast especially if you have binged on food and drinks over the previous days, while partying or during celebrations. During fasting, your body learns how to be efficient, and it uses some of the excess food in your system that you do not need. Do not eat just because the clock indicates it's time for a meal. Eat because you are hungry. The time between meals is not etched in stone; it varies between people, need, and activity level. If you have not lifted a finger all day, you probably do not need to eat more than enough to cover your BMR.

If you ate a large meal but are still hungry, maybe all you need is a nap, not a snack. Good sleep could be a remedy for ravenousness in two ways: it decreases the awake time allotted to eating, and it recharges the body on a physiological level. Very often, people mistake sleep deprivation and fatigue for hunger.

Before you reach for that soda or cheesecake, ask yourself whether what you are feeling is hunger or sleep deprivation. A minimum of six hours of good sleep each day may be the magic number of sleep hours we need. A good sleep usually harmonizes the synchronicity between the physical body and the mental realm. Failure to bring these two body energies together in harmony could result in dissociation, where the mind and body speak with divergent voices.

In addition to sleep, relaxation, rest, leisure, vacation, walking, meditation, and exercise can achieve harmony between the body and the mind, albeit in lesser degrees.

Make parts of the edible plant your diet pal

Many parts of plants are edible. During photosynthesis, plants convert carbon dioxide to carbohydrates. These carbohydrates are stored in parts of plants such as fruits, seeds, leafy vegetables, and edible plant-root tubers such as potatoes, carrots, and beets.

A common mistake people make while trying to lose weight is to eat nature's food in addition to junk food. Such an eating habit will do no one any good. I hear this all the time when I inquire about what kind of drinks people take. The answer is usually "Soda, but I also drink water." When I get that kind of feedback, I usually take some time to make myself clearer. My recommendation is for people to drink only ordinary, nonflavored water—not water in addition to soda but water in place of soda and Gatorade and all other soft drinks.

Fortunately, you do not have to be on the verge of catastrophe before you discover the importance of healthy eating. It is good to start eating healthily when young. Do not miss the opportunity to introduce children to healthy eating habits. Serve vegetables, fruits, and grains. Do not expose children to soda and refined sugar. I was not visionary enough to do that for my children, even though I was a doctor before they were born. The target is to make healthy eating a habit for children so that the fundamentals are there as they grow into adult life.

I will readily admit that it is impossible to win in all areas in the battle of healthy food choices. There are bound to be residual bad habits that you will be unable to shake. How I wish that I could replace my beloved early morning cup of coffee with a cool glass of water.

Exercise

Exercise is the other vital component in weight management. Nutritious food is the foundation to weight management, and exercise is an adjunct. Relying on exercise alone as a weight-control vehicle is short-sighted. It is bound to fail, because the body wanes in strength as people get older. Spirited, regular exercise ensures that all parts of the body are aerated and permeated with the nutrients they need for optimal body function.

Exercise activities can be divided into aerobic (in the presence of oxygen) and anaerobic (in the absence of oxygen). In a typical aerobic exercise such as walking, you are comfortable in breathing and exertion. In anaerobic exercise, such as sprinting up the hill, bicycling, or doing spirited dance moves, you exert a tremendous amount of muscle force and are visibly out of breath and physiologically out of proper muscle tissue oxygenation. Since the anaerobic type of exercise is more forceful, it burns more calories—but at the expense of muscle aches and shorter duration. The aerobic type of exercise is the more enduring exercise, but it burns fewer calories. The most serious exercise is a mix of the two, comprising both aerobic and anaerobic. This ensures that you recover in the aerobic phase after an intense anaerobic period.

Exercise choices must be carried out as tolerated. Otherwise, you may suffer a skeletal injury. Do not dunk a basketball if you are a sixty-five-year-old man. There are many varieties of exercise activities to choose from. Don't engage in rock climbing if you have an achy knee joint. Exercise activities can be a whole-body exercise, where you work up the entire body simultaneously, as in dancing and soccer, or a focused type of exercise, where you target an out-of-shape area such as the belly or the legs. I like to do a general type of body exercise. You can decide whether to exercise alone or as part of a group. I like to work out alone, as it provides me a quiet moment to think and reflect on life.

Go all the way

I met a friend at a local store recently. He had doubled in size since I'd last seen him, and I told him so. "But I exercise every day," he countered. But then he continued, "I love to eat my pounded cassava three times a day with melon soup." I suspected that he realized that the reason why his exercise was not making a difference in his weight was because he ate too much carbohydrate.

Begin your exercise activities today. Do not be plagued by excuses. It is natural for people to find excuses as to why they can't get things done. The truth is that we always find time to do the things we value most. Unconsciously, we rank our to-do list in order of importance.

Placing exercise activity at the bottom of the list is a mistake. It should come up after food, work, and rest. A lot is riding on our health, and exercise is an important part of it.

Exercise is one of those time-tested activities that is vital to humans. I have no doubt that nothing beats good exercise. It shakes off the cobwebs and brings the body out of doldrums. When you exercise, your metabolism will get sharper and your fat cells will shrivel.

My exercise preparation is simple. I put on my jeans and T-shirt, wear a sweatshirt over my T-shirt if the weather is cold, and put on my face cap and my sneakers. I make sure that my basketball is ready to go and get a bottle of water or a large cup of black coffee with no sugar. Then off I go. I usually ask my kids to come with me. It is a pleasure if they do, but I am all right if they do not. On weekends, I like to exercise in the mornings before most people wake up. On Wednesdays, I exercise in the evening when I get home from work. To accommodate my Wednesday exercise, I close my practice early, at about one thirty. I spend between ninety minutes and two hours from preparation to completion of exercise. I endeavor to do twice-a-week exercise activities.

Focus on problem areas, especially depending on your habits and body type. My lower extremities have remained trim because I am quick on my legs as a walker and a soccer player. To focus on my broad and chunky shoulders, I had to learn how to play basketball. In a ninety-minute session, which I do twice a week, I throw about three hundred shots. Now my scapula is as flat as a plank, and I have built good upper-muscle strength. Some people may want to work on different parts of their bodies. The good news is that fat will be flushed out from wherever it resides when you lose general body weight.

Cerebellum and movement coordination

The cerebellum, part of the hind brain, participates a great deal in body movement coordination. A great deal of coordination goes on in the brain to get your feet or hands to move in a timely fashion when you need them and on target where you want them. Your cerebellum is in the middle of it all, overseeing your limbs and ensuring that your body obeys your movement desires in a prompt and decisive manner. The capability to walk heel to toe is among some of the movement skills that are made possible by cerebellum coordination. I use heel-to-toe walking, controlled pacing, and linear alignment as ways to fire up my cerebellum connections.

A lot more people engage in walking as part of their exercise menu than perhaps any other form of exercise. Walking is such an inveterate human activity. A lot can be accomplished with walking. You can walk fast or slow. I find it productive and exhilarating to tweak my walks.

Make your walk exciting by adding variations to it. Some people like to walk with weights attached to their arms or legs. I do not like to do that because it slows me down. Be sure that the variety of walk you choose suits your peculiar physical and health condition. Avoid all environmental hazards prior to trying out the techniques. I do not advocate that people walk on roads. My various walking techniques include the following:

- walking backward
- walking in a straight line
- walking down a slope
- walking up a hill
- walking sideways
- heel-to-toe walking

Lots of ideas come during exercise activities. This is my second book in a year. I am fired up. I credit the surge in my creative thinking and writing to my activities and plant-based nutrition. By increasing the body's blood flow, nutrients, and oxygen supplies, exercise undoubtedly invigorates and rejuvenates body tissues.

Facial fat fades in conjunction with general body fat and vice versa. Many people are concerned with the appearance of their faces—the numerous facial products on the market give evidence to that. We want to present our best face to the world. The face is a window through which others look into our emotion. When we are sad or happy, it shows in our face.

Facial exercise and massage is easily accomplished while taking a shower. My favorite technique is to support my entire lower jaw on my two thumbs and part of my palm and then fan out my other eight fingers across my face, my cheek, and below my lower eyelid for deep strokes and massage. The best time to do this is at the end of your shower. I usually spend two to three minutes doing this massage.

The human brain—the human cerebral cortex—is made up of two halves, the cerebral hemispheres. For most people, the right side of the brain controls the left side of their body, and vice versa. About 90 percent of people are right-hand dominant, which means they are controlled by their left cerebral hemisphere. Part of my regular exercise is to temporarily reverse that setup. For about fifteen minutes, I do all my shooting baskets and rebound activities with my nondominant left hand and left leg. My intention is to strengthen the muscle groups in that half region of my body, which otherwise will not get as much regular shooting actions as my dominant half. The added hope is to also ignite my nondominant right cerebral hemisphere, benefiting from any of its subtle functional difference.

Use what you already have

You do not need to buy extravagant and expensive equipment just because you want to lose weight. Find something that you already have at home. The same idea applies to location. You do not need to waste money on a monthly membership to a fitness center. Start with a public park or a local high school. Your backyard also is a good place to begin, if you have one. Also, do not waste your money on designer-food delivery. Make your own food; it is easy when you think of natural food. I incurred minimal cost when I started on my weight-loss regimen. I only had to buy a new basketball. I retrieved a pair of sneakers from the garage.

Playing basketball is my main exercise preference, even though I did not play as a kid. I got better as I played more. Each of my sessions lasts for about ninety minutes. I endeavor to shoot up to three hundred times from the three-point range. I do jump-shots. I run to catch rebounds. I shoot with my left hand. Initially, I was well off the mark—lots of air balls. But I kept practicing, and later good things began to happen to me on the court. My shots began to fall into the basket. I improved my three-point shots from a 10 percent shooter to a 20 percent shooter, unguarded. The rim became friendlier. I began to make good on some awkward shots, including many half-court shots. I also made many shots outside the arc, using my leg.

My exercise time serves both as a meditation moment and a physical activity time. Chasing the bouncing ball gives me the opportunity to work my upper body, my lower body, and my shoulders. I rebound, catch, throw, sprint, and walk on the court. It is a total workup of aerobic and anaerobic exercise.

Try whatever works for you. If working out with fitness tapes or DVDs helps with your exercise, stay on it—but you have to participate. Do not just be an onlooker. Watching a tape or DVD will not make you lose weight; participating will. I did not know about Zumba until I attended a Zumba fund-raising event organized by my daughter Amy and led by Miss Taylor of Newtown Youth Center. For an hour we danced to a variety of music. It was fun.

Check out your local schools and parks. Form an informal walking group, running group, or dancing group with your neighbors and friends. Look for a free or low-cost gym. If your town does not have an adequate park, check a neighboring town.

Examples of exercise outlets
- outdoors—fields and parks
- indoors, at home
- groups such as Zumba
- job-organized walk
- gym

Choose an exercise environment that is safe and secure. Running on a busy road or walking alone on a lonely trail is probably not a very good idea.

Disease conditions

Acute or chronic disease can act up at any time during or after exercise. Staying ahead of what could go wrong is very essential.

Osgood-Schlatter disease, or OSD, is a common knee problem in young adults and youths. It is a soreness of the top of the tibia bone where it connects with the quadriceps tendon, below the kneecap. Treatment of this condition includes rest, local analgesic, and warm compresses on the affected knee.

If you suffer from asthma, be sure to have your asthma pump with you during exercise. You might need it before and during exercise activity, especially if you are outdoors. I have seen kids with asthma panting while they are playing basketball. This could get dangerous. If this happens, stop playing and get immediate medical help.

Backache may be a sign of an unstable vertebral disc and a warning of impending disc prolapse. Stop the exercise until you see a doctor. A chest pain during exercise could be a sign of compromised blood flow to the heart. Stop the activities until you are properly cleared by a doctor. If you hit your head on the floor, or if you got hit on the head by an object, it might be a good time to call it quits until you are fully evaluated for concussion.

Carry a bottle or two of cold water along with you, especially in hot weather. Though some parks have vending machines, a bottle of water will cost almost double the normal price. Some parks have water fountains, but sanitation may be an issue.

Try not to injure yourself. Follow all the recommended safety precautions. Wear a helmet if you are riding a bicycle. Do not play basketball on a wet court. Go home if the park is closed—it is closed for a reason. Survey your environment before any sport activities. Remove potentially dangerous materials from your field.

CHAPTER 9

Stay the Course

Changing ingrained habits such as diet and activity lifestyle is not as hard as it seems. This last chapter will provide you with the tips and assurance you need to easily implement the strategies recommended in this book. Everything about dieting starts with a firm commitment.

Commitment is not lip service of "I will," which is what many people do as a New Year's resolution. It is a conscious process based on a complete understanding of why you have undertaken the new path, as well as determination to carry it out. For it to work, a person has to value the reasons why a change in nutrition lifestyle is important.

Commitment strategies
1. Recognize the importance and the urgency of the needed changes.
2. Begin with baby-step changes, both in nutrition and physical activities.
3. Anticipate obstacles.
4. Be ready to redo and recharge your focus.
5. Stay with your program.
6. Learn what works and what doesn't work.
7. Learn from the mistakes and successes of others.
8. Continue self-education.
9. Embrace your success.

10. Make it a habit.

Give yourself a chance

The mind can be our greatest obstacle to commitment. Do not let your mind talk you into quitting prematurely. The key to weight loss is not dissimilar to other aspirations—you must give yourself a chance. Do not abandon your strategy when you encounter a setback. If Barack Obama had done that, he wouldn't have become president. Get back on it. Obstacles are to be expected. More obstacles exist in this arena, perhaps, than in any other individual endeavor.

There is always a general malaise around weight management, based on the supposition that though the mind is willing, the body is weak. I beg to differ; the body is not weak. Our body obediently adapts to the wishes of our mind.

I did not think that I was capable of making the changes myself, but it became easier once I got past the first few days and weeks. People tend to stay on the things that benefit them, the things that they consider necessary. Going to work is a necessity for obvious reasons, so people tend to stay in their jobs for decades or even for a lifetime. Change always boils down to what we want to fight for and what we want to give up.

Dieting, good nutrition, and exercise deserve better attention in our lives than many of us give them. The good news is that if you commit to the changes, your body will take care of the rest. The physiological changes that go with neuroplasticity and cellular adaptation are deep and demonstrable in the cellular chemistry.

Many of us don't rush to gulp down pain pills each time we feel an ache. We wait, hoping that the hurt will go away, which is what happens most of the time. NBA players get stomped on their toes and ankles very frequently. They do not swig down Tylenol or Advil or Aleve each time that happens. They walk it off. Their pain goes away in no time. So why would you rush to eat each time you experience what could well be a false hunger pang

Learn to maintain some control. Restrain yourself until the hunger feeling is established. Everybody needs to practice how to fill their void with awareness and introspection, rather than with food and drinks.

Humans are a bundle of nerves. Our emotions run wild in many directions. We are hardly in control of our thoughts, our emotions, or our appetite. Delaying gratification is a practice that we need to learn. Give that wine enough time to cool in the fridge before you drink it. Let the soup cook before you devour it. Learn to wait to be served. Do not rush to the food store for any false sign of hunger.

Active, not a passive process

The notion that one can medicate oneself into weight loss does not pass a common-sense test. Taking pills daily over a long period of time for weight control is not a good idea because of potential side effects. Lifestyle changes must be part of any sustainable weight-loss effort.

Having a "sweet tooth" is a myth. When people say they have a sweet tooth, they are probably referring to hyperfunctioning sugar taste buds on their tongue. If you love sweets, your normal taste buds will balloon in size to accommodate your sweet desire. Remember, added sugar is implicated in the epidemic of type 2 diabetes. Nobody is born with a sweet tooth; it is developed. And because we develop a sweet tooth, we can make it go away. This leads me to the biological concept of cell adaptation.

Think of cell adaptation as your body cells stepping up to the plate, to meet with your demand, and retreating when they are no longer in need. For example, if you are training hard to compete in a sprint, your calf muscle cells may increase in size to prepare you for the competition. After the race, when you no longer are in training, your calf muscle cells will retreat to their original size and numbers. Next year, if you need them, you may have to train as hard as before to get them to their winning sizes again.

Similarly, when you crave and eat sugary food, your taste buds will proliferate to deal with the sugar. You now have "sweet tooth." Conversely, when you work hard to get rid of your sweet tooth, your sweet taste buds will adapt and become less intrusive and less noticeable—and may, in fact, disappear. This is why you may not enjoy your favorite delicacy with the same savor that you had after you stopped eating it for a time.

Likewise, people who are accustomed to smaller meals tend to possess smaller stomach capacity; it fits the size of the meals they eat. That is why people may feel nauseated when they take on a meal portion larger than what they normally eat. If they get used to larger portions of meals, however, their stomach capacity will eventually yield to accommodate their desire.

Some people feel they will never get used to nature's own food because they think it does not taste as good or smell as good as processed food. Obviously, they underestimate the wonders of the human brain and neuroplasticity.

Neuroplasticity is the capability of the brain neuron to be malleable and rewire. The brain, which is the seat of wisdom, has billions of neurons that ensure signal communication between parts of the body. Our sensual perception of smell, taste, sight, touch, and hearing depends on the manner in which neurons link up with themselves and their impulse trajectory across involved areas of the nervous system.

Very frequently, the brain neurons have to redo their interconnection patterns to accommodate new, learned behaviors. Do not worry about how your taste buds will react to your new and improved food choices. In due course, you will get used to nature's own aroma.

Months ago, my son told me of an occasion when he and his friend made tea. While he completed his tea, pouring in packets of sugar, his friend was enjoying his own tea equally well without sugar. My son was dumbfounded and inquired if his friend had forgotten to add sugar. "Not at all," his friend said. "I do not use sugar for my tea." In my practice, I know of children who would never eat cereal when it contains sugar. They will never do it, because they were never introduced to it.

As with many endeavors you will encounter naysayers. These are people who know and understand but are not ready to give up their bad food habits and inactivity. They will tell you that they know people who smoked until they were ninety years old. They will say they know people who ate all they wanted and never went to see a doctor. They know somebody who was as lean as a rake, adhered to a diet of vegetables, whole grains, milk, and fruits, yet were stricken with one disease after another. They might be right. But these individuals do not conform to the average.

Educate yourself and explore the world of plant-based food

A good part of weight maintenance is continual education and learning from other people's experiences. Make valuing and appreciating the immense diversity and availability of plant-based food the core of your learning.

My favorite time while writing this book was when I went to stores to find the fruits, nuts, and vegetables that I read about in the books but had never seen. It was like making a new friend. I got to look, touch, feel, and interact with other realms of nature's own creation. It is fulfilling. I was so excited when I saw soybeans for the first time. How could I have lived fifty years without getting to know sunflower seeds, for instance, or almonds, Brazil nuts, squash, and so forth?

Stay tuned to the latest information on food and nutrition. This is a rapidly expanding and evolving area, with lots of revisions and recommendations based on ongoing science and observation. Research the food and snacks or beverages you consume, especially those that you consume frequently. You can find useful information about food online. For example, if you like peanuts, like I do, Google it to find its nutrients and composition.

Drive around your neighborhood to find shops, or ask your friends and family about stores and food outlets that carry food that suits your new and improved nutritional lifestyle. Identify and buy from outlets that sell healthy, fresh produce. There should be some in your neighborhood.

Relying on your doctor to tell you how your health issues are related to your food choices and activity lifestyle may not materialize effortlessly. Some doctors don't bother with patients' nutrition because they do not get adequately reimbursed for doing that. It may take hours of time to evaluate a person's food and nutritional habits and social lifestyle and then offer needed counseling and management. Besides, there is no guarantee that the session will be fruitful once the patient leaves the office. In addition, many doctors are not knowledgeable in nutrition matters. Physicians hardly get any in-depth education during medical school about food, cooking, and the varieties of food available.

Hang with the optimists

If you want to be a good dancer, you hang with the dancers, and if you want to be a scholar, you hang with the professors. In the same manner, if you want to eat healthily, go to lunch and dinner with folks who eat healthily. Do not bother with the cynics. They will forecast that you will give up, give in, and quit in six months or one year. They will give you lists of real people who have since abandoned the road to healthy eating. They will cajole you to come back to the tent of cheesecake crunchers, hot-dog devourers, cookie monsters, and fried-chicken whoppers.

Chose nature's own diet above exercise

Exercise without proper diet is like prayer without faith. You will never pass a fitness test doing that. Don't think that you can eat all you want because you work it out later. It never works out right. It is not a good idea to gulp a cheeseburger because you have a soccer game in the evening. The same applies to a chocolate bar or doughnuts. You will be left with pounds under your belt. If you were to choose between eating healthily and exercise, chose the former all the time.

The mistake people frequently make is thinking that they can eat all the junk they want because they will be going to the gym. The problem is that most times, that next exercise engagement never comes at all, or when it comes, it frequently falls short of the desired result. It is easier to load up on calories but harder to get rid of them. Let us look at the logistics of loading up and burning.

A series of events once conspired to deny me my routine exercise sessions. First, my daughter had to be taken for a learner's permit exam on a Saturday morning, and then on the following Saturday, she missed her bus to a school event, which meant that I had to drop her and pick her up. Then, the following Saturday, she was so sick that my exercise time was put on hold. Then there was a snowstorm that shut down every exercise outlet. Surprisingly, my weight did not change during these periods. What saved me was very simple: I ate healthily. I stuck to my usual natural food.

People tend to eat more when they are idle. Be engaged when at home and at work. Sitting in front of the television frequently goes with a bottle of beer or chips or snacks. Do not be a sitting duck. Read a book or a magazine. Help your kids with their homework. Call your friend for a chat. Get yourself outdoors—garden or rake leaves. Knit, sew, or volunteer at a local community church or event.

Avoid taking food, snacks, or drinks with you to the bedroom. Adults do not need a nighttime snack. In addition, our digestive system slows down at night when we are supposed to be sleeping. Eat all you desire in the kitchen, wash your hands, and leave.

Often we mistake exhaustion, fatigue, boredom, sorrow, restlessness, impatience, and insomnia for hunger and then proceed to fill the bottomless emptiness with junk food.

I thought I was hungry, but when I woke up after a good sleep, my hunger disappeared. I was looking for something to eat from the fridge but got sidetracked when I got a call from an old friend. We ended up talking for one hour. When we finished talking I was so excited, I went out with my children to the movies. Everybody probably has a story like that—or vice versa, when they ate chips because nobody was home to engage them in a friendly discussion.

Learn how to stop and think. Are you really hungry? When was the last time you ate? Has it been long enough that you ought to be hungry at this moment? If the answer is no, you are probably not hungry and need to divert your attention from food.

The "tangible intangibles" are things that look tiny but make a huge impact, one way or the other, when summed up. I stumbled on a packet of flavored French vanilla cream in my kitchen. I read the label: one small container had 30 calories and contained 5 grams of sugar. If I were to pour in five of those packets in a cup of tea, I would give myself 150 empty sugar calories. You can choose to avoid that by using nonflavored milk instead. Or use one or two flavored packets instead of five.

If you must indulge in a sandwich with fried egg, do not let oil dribble all over your sandwich like a mini waterfall. You can dramatically cut the quantity of oil you use—and the calories from oil—by investing in a nonstick frying pan. My preference is a boiled egg sandwich, rather than a fried egg sandwich.

Search for and use nature's own spices. There are flavors in grains, in nuts, in pepper, in onions, in vegetables, in fresh milk, in fruits, in seeds, in tomatoes, in avocados, and so forth. You also can spice food with natural spices, such as thyme, parsley, oregano, or cinnamon.

The good news is, if you give nature's own food flavors a chance, you will grow to love them.

Between the months of June and September 2012, I did a random collection of height and weight of thirty-two children, ages six to ten, that I saw in my medical office. The children were both male and female, mostly of black and Hispanic background. I then looked up their BMI from a standard BMI chart on my office wall. During the routine encounter, I asked their mothers, "What does your child usually eat for breakfast? What is his favorite meal for breakfast?" This gave me a specific identification—for example, that the child liked only chocolate cereal. Some of the kids ate from only one food category (e.g., boxed cereals); others ate from a mix of assorted food groups.

Below is a sample of the raw data:

Age	BMI	Breakfast	Mom's comment
6	15.5	None	Wakes up late
6	16	French toast	Picky eater
6	18	Oatmeal, egg	
6	29, abnormal	Boxed cereals	Cocoa Puffs
6	16	Eggs, plantain, oatmeal	
6	15.5	Watermelon, yogurt	

7	16	Scrambled egg and pancake	
7	15	Salad, bacon	Active
7	16	Oatmeal, waffle	
7	21, abnormal	Sandwich: ham, egg, and cheese	
7	16	Oatmeal	Yet to eat breakfast at noon
7	17	Hash browns	Picky eater
8	16	Bagel and cream cheese	
8	20	Cheese and bagel	
8	15	Bacon, egg, cheese	Likes to exercise
8	24, abnormal	Waffles, cereals	
8	16.6	Cereal, sausage, eggs	Active, runs a lot
8	19	Cereals	Cereal, mostly
8	28, abnormal	Cookie cereals	
8	14	Vegetarian	Picky eater
9	21.5	Pancake, cereals	Chocolate cereals
9	17	Fish, beans, rice	
9	24.5, abnormal	Ham, cheese, and pancake	
9	15	Cereal, Frosted Flakes	Picky eater
9	15	Varies	Yet to eat breakfast at 1 p.m.
9	17	Ham, egg, sandwich	
10	23	French toast, juice	
10	26.5, abnormal	Peanut butter sandwich	

10	24, abnormal	Eggs, bacon, or waffles	
10	22	Boxed cereal	
10	17.5	Sandwich: egg and cheese	Picky eater
10	13, underweight	Picky eater	Avoids food due to food allergies

Other factors might contribute to the nature of data presented above, but the principal conclusion is that the kids who had normal BMI not only ate healthier and had a more active lifestyle, but they were also picky eaters.

Attend community health fair

Attend a local health fair in your community when you can. You will be amazed by the wisdom you gain from individuals and collective experience. You may learn more from a session like this than you will by yourself in months or in a lifetime.

I had plenty to learn when I attended one of the local health fairs. The event was organized by the Bridgeport Chamber of Commerce. The panelists gave their prepared speeches, after which there was an open dialogue with the audience.

What I learned from the panel

Recognition of the need to change course is the easy part in dieting. The hard part, the panelists reiterated, was to commit to the required change. The audience identified some of the obstacles to weight maintenance: time constraints, stress, and life in the fast lane.

One panelist advocated using the 4/7/8 breathing/relaxation technique as a way to combat stress and stress eating. Breathe in for four seconds, hold the breath for seven seconds, and exhale over eight seconds.

Other suggestions by the panel included:

- Write down your goals and what you want to achieve: fitness, weight loss, muscle tone, good looks, younger body, getting healthy.
- Identify and connect to available resources around you. Ask your friends and neighbors.
- Monitor and measure your progress periodically.
- Celebrate your success. It may encourage others to emulate your victory and follow in your footsteps.
- Join support and enhancement groups.
- Getting your family to join and share in your effort may have a sustaining effect.
- If you are sincere about your effort, you will be more likely to succeed.
- It is hard to go back to your old eating habits once you succeed in breaking them.
- Share information on what works and what doesn't.
- How you deliver your message as a healthy diet advocate is as important as the message.

Will junk food go the way of the cigarette?

During the floor discussion, one of the attendees reminded the audience that cigarette smoking has vanished from most homes just in a span of ten years. He predicted that if we apply the same focus to nutrition, the tide might turn against junk food and the junk-food industry. Watch out, junk food—you may go the way of the cigarette.

If you can identify foods in their natural forms, you can make yourself a good meal. Recipes evolve from the depths of human tastes. Be critical of them. Lots of diet recipes are detours back to the exaggerated taste buds of high and empty calories, which are what weight watchers are trying to run away from.

Recipes are indigenous. Within any given country, recipes still vary from ethnicity to ethnicity. It is not hard to imagine that many recipes may have started as healthy but along the journey of time, some of them became unwholesome. One must learn how to dissect and evaluate a recipe.

Food recipes, however, are overrated. The steps are often numerous and their ingredients frequently are unnecessary. Recipes will sway you to add sugar or syrup; to pour in this wine or that oil; to sprinkle in salt or sugar; to throw in more butter or add cheese. Most of these additives are needless. Overstuffed recipes are a hindrance to healthy eating. In the end, people have succeeded in turning nature's own food into a bad meal. The same thing was echoed by Dr. Oz in a CNN interview with Piers Morgan. He said that though coffee is an antioxidant, the problem is that what started off as coffee has quickly turned into a chocolate bar by the addition of lots of sugar and cream.

Below is a version of a yam porridge recipe from Igbo, Nigeria.

My mother or sisters would peel the skin off cut yams. The yams were then thrown into a pot and cooked until their entire thickness was softened. Then Mother would add lots of vegetables, ground pepper, onions, crayfish, palm oil, and salt. She continued to cook and stir until all the yams were stuck within the mixture. Since there was no automated grinder, the pepper, crayfish, and onions were crushed to a pulp in a wooden mortar with a wooden pestle. The porridge was served in bowls and eaten with hands, forks, or spoons.

Ingredients
- yam
- vegetables
- crayfish
- water
- palm oil
- pepper
- salt

My version of the above recipe has no salt or oil. All other ingredients are the same. The point is to be able to recognize a recipe that is inadequate, based on current knowledge and observation, and try to fix it.

Why not make up your own recipe as I do. On this day, I was scheduled to work in the morning. When I woke up at five in the morning, I poured some lentils into a pot that was half-full of water and began to heat it up. In a separate pot, I put in some spinach and water and turned on the stove. Then I went to take a bath and shave. About fifteen minutes later, my vegetables were done. In about forty-five minutes, my lentils were done. I packed them for work. I love to eat spinach and lentils simultaneously. My drink was a large cup of black coffee. I used four small, nonflavored half-and-half milk cups. That was what I had for breakfast and dinner. What a delicious meal! I chose lentils because they cook in a shorter time. One can select from any of the other grains. Grains and vegetables are packed with nutrients, antioxidants, proteins, minerals, carbohydrates, and fibers. I did not need salt. I did not need sugar. I did not need oil.

Nature-based recipes

First, select what you would like to eat from among nature's major food groups: grains, legumes, plant-derived carbohydrates, fish.

Have some onions, tomatoes, peppers, leafy vegetables, or seeds to go with your meal.

- Examples of grains are oat, wheat, or brown rice.
- Examples of legumes are beans, lentils, or peas.
- Examples of plant-derived carbohydrates are potato, yam, and yucca, also known as cassava.
- Examples of leafy vegetables are broccoli, spinach, celery, and chicory.

Two pots will be ideal but one pot will do as well. Start by setting up the components of your main food materials. For example, rewash your grain or your lentils. Peel the skin off your yam or potato if you need to. Cut your onions and peppers. You may also want to wash and cut your vegetables and get them ready.

Boil your grain or legume or yam until cooked or almost done. Add water repeatedly, as needed, to get it softened. Grains and legumes may triple in size during cooking, so allow room in your pot for your grains to swell.

It is useful to know the estimated cooking time of your main food. Legumes such as beans can take about ninety minutes to cook, while lentils and peas can be softened in half the time. Another downside to beans is that they may make you flatulent. You can diminish this by putting in fresh water as they cook. Figuring out the time your main food is done is easy. Scoop a small amount of grain in a spoon during cooking to determine whether it is soft enough. Be careful not to burn your tongue. Then add your onions and peppers, and continue cooking for another five minutes. Last, add your cut vegetables and allow them to simmer with the rest of the food for an extra five minutes. Then you are ready to eat.

You can also elect to cook the vegetables separately; add a little bit of water to onions, tomatoes, and peppers, followed by the main vegetable. You can sprinkle in a teaspoon of your favorite seeds, such as flaxseed. When done, your meal will have flavors—the real type of flavors, which are the natural flavors.

My favorite soup recipe
I try to prepare this soup twice weekly, on Wednesday for dinner and on Saturday for lunch.

Ingredients
- tomatoes, sliced tomato
- onions, cut onion
- spinach, cut spinach
- broccoli
- coconuts, cut coconut
- pepper/hot pepper

Preparation of my soup recipe
I use about four medium fresh tomatoes and two medium onions. I slice both into chunks and put them in a pot containing about two cups of

water. Then I cook them until they soften up. That takes ten to fifteen minutes. Next into the pot is my mixture of cut hot peppers, spinach, and broccoli. To finish up the soup, I pour in my harvest-fresh coconut water. I usually allow the broth to cook together for another five minutes before I turn off the stove.

For more details on recipes and calorie counts, check out Harvard School of Public Health's Nutrition Source (http://www.hsph.harvard.edu/nutritionsource/).

Reasons why people relapse after weight loss

Relapse in weight loss occurs when someone goes back to the bad, old food habits and inactivity previously conquered. People can relapse in a matter of days or months or years. Relapse could be a result of several factors. It may be as whimsical as a new friend or relative coming to town. An old friend or a relative in town may sway someone to change his or her eating habits to accommodate the friend.

When my sister visited from Nigeria, I gained five pounds in one week. This was because my sister introduced her Nigerian method of food preparation, which includes lots of condiments.

Flavor is the hallmark of a well-prepared African food. With the flavor, however, comes the addition of unwanted pounds of weight. Though my sister's food was delicious, I had to change course quickly. I told her how I liked my food prepared. I like the flavors in my food to come from natural plants. Every plant has its natural, unadulterated flavor, and I like sticking with that. She listened, and the five pounds of extra weight quickly evaporated.

Some of the more deep-rooted reasons for regaining lost weight could be

- incomplete resolution of weight problem,
- partial or total lack of understanding of issues relating to problems,
- lack of understanding,
- commitment abandonment,

- loss of support,
- return of old stressors, and
- encounter with new stressors.

In addition to the total social breakdown enumerated above, there could be a biological explanation of why people regain weight after weight loss. This hypothesis is based solely on my observations.

During the long period of weight loss, the body cells get used to operating on a low carbohydrate environment. Any increase in calories to prior quantity is met with immediate conversion of the excess calories to fat, which is then stored in the body, contributing to rapid weight gain. This theory is in keeping with the body's way of functioning, which is to mainly use carbohydrates as fuel and fat as a storage medium of choice. This hypothesis also fits with the recognition that most of the body's weight fluctuation is due to its fat component. If someone totally abandons all nutritional commitment, he or she reaches an equilibrium, where body cells adjust and weight gain becomes less dramatic.

Relapse-buster tips

- RENEW YOUR VOW DAILY, NOT YEARLY.

When challenges come, remember your motivations. Fight back; remember what motivated you. Recalling what motivated your journey is a good way to stay focused. Many times, it is a peculiar event in our lives that stops all the vacillation on what we need to do and jolts us into decisive action. It could be a minor health scare, like I had in 2010, or it could be a major health scare, like President Clinton had. In 2004, former president Clinton suffered blocked coronary arteries and had to undergo bypass surgery. Leading to that incident, Clinton had indulged in unhealthy food habits. He loved fast-food, fries, nuggets, and soft drinks. Since his ordeal, the former president has eaten healthier and exercised more frequently. He is committed to healthy nutrition and lifestyle. He kicked the fast-food habit.

The so-called executive region of the brain is located in the frontal cortex area of the cereberal hemisphere. It is the area of the brain mostly responsible for impulse control, decision making, and behavioral management. For example, the question of whether to use the bathroom now or later is adjudicated by the executive region of the brain. Similarly, the question of whether to eat now or eat later is also decided by this area of the brain.

Eating and weight fluctuation is a struggle between hunger and satiety. At the most basic level, a person will eat only when he or she feels hungry and will stop when he or she is satiated. This primordial sense of control is at the autonomic level, which is that part of the central nervous functioning regardless of our input. The autonomic feeding thermostat is precise in newborns. They wake up every two hours or so to feed. Once they are full, they will refuse to eat until the next feeding cycle. As people get older, this rhythmic biological clock, the hypothalamus, becomes crusted by the demands of social pressure around us, to the extent that we can no longer accurately tell when we are hungry or when we are not.

There are two main hormones at play during the hunger and satiety signals in the body. The hormone *ghrelin* sends signals to some areas of the hypothalamus that we are hungry. In response, we seek food. The signal to stop when full is provided by, among other factors, a hormone called *leptin*. This hormone is produced by body fat tissues.

Hence, to eat or not to eat is prompted by the body physiological mechanism, but ultimately, it's under the supervision of the body's executive approval. How the executive decision is made often determines how we control our appetite and what and when we eat.

The executive brain—not so executive

The word *executive* sounds so dependable, you would think that the executive brain makes firm decisions all the time. It does not. The executive part of the brain is like a company executive who is expected to make the right decisions at all times. But in reality, each day the company executive is swarmed by a variety of internal and external factors that inhibit wise judgment and actions. Subtle internal factors, such as temperament, emotions, money, choices, and information can have a tremendous effect on executive decisions.

Likewise, the human executive has to deal with input from hundreds of billions of neurons, all carrying their own sways. The impulse, be it from food flavors, memory, sight, touch, or music, are trying to influence the executive decision making.

Tips to tame your executive brain
1. Surround yourself with nutritious food, so that even when you give in, you are eating good and nutritious food.
2. Avoid exposure to junk and processed food.
3. Say no to junk and processed food.

To end this book, I will give you what I consider to be my one-minute pitch on helping you contain your weight so that you can stay healthy. Stay away from sodas and soft drinks of any kind. And if you want to do more, do not eat any shelf item with more than one gram of added sugar. Do not taint nature's food with fat, fried oil, and salt.

Recommendations
Estimate your BMI and daily calorie need, based on your activity level. Target eliminating five hundred calories per week. This should be easy by following the guidelines below. Please check with your clinician if you are in doubt or have any contraindicated medical conditions.

1. Diversify among the major food groups.
2. Know your BMI; stay in the normal range.
3. Replace meat protein with plant protein.
4. Eat lots of vegetables, and eat a moderate amount of fruits.
5. Devote 90–120 minutes, twice a week, for vigorous physical activities.
6. Tweak your exercise activities.
7. Nature's own diet beats exercise at all times.

8. Too much of good food is equally as bad as unhealthy food.
9. Do not buy shelf food with more than one gram of sugar in it.
10. Fast or skip a meal when you are not hungry.
11. Be wary of all snacks; they add up.
12. Eat small quantities at a time.
13. Try new food; you don't know what you are missing.
14. Buy only from the produce areas of the store.
15. Take time to make your own meals.
16. Eat baked, not fried, foods.
17. Kiss all soft drinks good-bye.
18. Eat only nature's own food—it took billions of years to perfect.
19. Check your weight twice weekly to determine where you are.
20. Research what you eat on the Internet.
21. Read labels; zero in on sugar content, fat, and salt.
22. Avoid added sugar at all costs and in all forms.
23. Limit salt to daily recommended amount—½ tsp.
24. Replace all bad food habits with good new food habits.
25. Target eliminating five hundred calories per week.

Test your understanding with this food puzzle

Qualities	Choices
1. May contain deadly doses of hydrogen cyanide	A. Unsaturated fat
	B. Celery
2. May contain aflatoxin	
	C. Contaminated tree nuts
3. Rich in lycopene	
	D. Tryptophan
4. Plant food with lots of saturated fat	
	E. Bitter almond
5. A vegetable with lots of sodium	
	F. Omega fatty acids
6. A grain with low quantity of vitamin B3, niacin	G. Palm kernel, coconuts, chocolate
7. Good natural source of iodine	H. Leafy vegetables
8. Part of the essential fatty acids	I. Tomato, watermelon
9. A legume with lots of fiber	J. Lentils
10. Culprit in obesity	K. Soda
11. Has minimal to no fat content	L. Trans fat
12. Legume with high fat content	M. Maize
13. Good fat	N. Soybean
14. Bad kind of fat	O. Lycopene
15. Good for prostate health	P. Table salt
16. Raises serotonin level and used in the treatment of insomnia and anxiety	Q. Kelp, eggs
	R. Turmeric
17. Only one teaspoon recommended per day	
18. Contains essential plant oil; used in curry	

Answer key is on next page:

1E, 2C, 3I, 4G, 5B, 6M, 7Q, 8F,
9J, 10K, 11H, 12N, 13A, 14L, 15O,
16D, 17P, 18R

Afterword

I like to call the first stage in weight loss the "shuffle stage," because that is when a dieter must expunge all of his or her bad eating habits and replace them with good eating habits. The shuffle stage is the most difficult stage. During this period, people battle the factors that come with lifestyle changes. Individual effort is sure to be challenged by self-doubt and internal and external factors. The goal in this stage is to halt further weight gain and give the body the time to unravel its fat deposit.

If you gain weight instead of losing, it means you may not be covering all the angles presented in this book. Successful completion of the first stage leads to the second stage, the momentum stage.

The momentum stage is the easiest stage, as the body would gladly give up lots of stored fat that it does not need. The rewards are tremendous. You will feel elated by your accomplishments. You may experience a surge of energy and vitality because of your choice of nature's own food. How many pounds you lose should depend on your BMI. The goal is to bring your BMI within its normal range for age and activity level. The amount you decide you to lose is an individual decision.

The third stage is the consolidation and equilibrium stage. During weight loss, a person's weight reaches equilibrium near the point where his or her BMI is normalized. My current weight of 153 pounds corresponds to a BMI of 23.8, which is within the normal range. The BMI must be treated as a reference guide, not an absolute number. You likely will bounce around near the equilibrium point. Weight maintenance for the long haul may be achieved by continuing all the suggestions learned in this book.

Glossary

basal metabolic rate (BMR): the energy your body needs to run its basic vital functions, such as heartbeat, digestion, kidney function, mental effort, etc.

body mass index (BMI): a measure of body fat based on height and weight. *ede*: the Igbos, Nigeria, word for cocoyam or malanga.

calorie: energy or fuel contained in a given food.

endocrine: a gland or tissue that secrets hormones.

exocrine: cells that release hormones or transmitters to the surrounding tissue.

hormones: chemical messengers in the body and bloodstream that cause physiological and biochemical changes. For example, insulin is a hormone secreted by the pancreas; insulin regulates blood sugar.

impulse: propagation of an action or signal from one body cell to another.

mpoto ede: the broad leaves of cocoyam. Do not hug; it is scratchy.

About the Author

This book was written from the perspective of a physician who solved his own weight challenges and has maintained normal weight for over two years. As a clinician in private practice, I am in that rank of endangered middle class who constantly fight the headwind of time, money, and family. With three children—ages twenty, sixteen, and thirteen—I think my life intersects in many ways with those of many Americans.

I was born in Nigeria, the fifth of ten children. I completed medical school at the university college hospital, Ibadan, Nigeria. In 1992, I immigrated to the United States. From 1993 to 1996, I did my residency program in pediatrics at Brookdale Hospital, Brooklyn, New York.

In rural Nigeria, where I grew up, there were lots of fruits to choose from. A typical neighborhood backyard had mango trees, peas, banana, pawpaw, pineapple, palms, wine trees, oranges, fresh corn, and guava. It sure was like the garden of Eden but without the divine constraint. Children ran around and ate from all the trees.

Facing the challenges of survival in urban New York City, I had to succumb to what was readily available and expedient: work, confinement, coffee, fast food, refined cereal, soda, chocolate bars, ice cream, and processed food. The weight piled up.

It took nearly twenty years and a looming catastrophe for me to catch my breath, to rediscover my life, to retool my lifestyle, to take responsibility for what I eat, to get back to the basics of what food should be, to redefine who I want to be based on what I eat, and to remember what my grandmother and mother taught me when they put a plate of food in front of me.

In this book, I brought forth my gift of being able to trim a complex subject down to the essentials.

Other books I have written are *Let the Dead Man Walk*, *Automated Man*, *Thought Inheritance*, and *The Cycle of Existence*.

References, Resources, and Details

Most of the references deal with the contemporary recommendations on food, nutrition, and physical activities. The topics overlap in content. Narrow down to the topics that interest you and educate yourself as much as you can.

Source:
"Food, nutrition, physical activity and the prevention of cancer—A global perspective." World Cancer Research Fund & American Institute for Cancer Research, 2007.

Source:
"Dietary Reference Intakes for Energy, Carbohydrate, Fiber, Fat, Fatty Acids, Cholesterol, Protein, and Amino Acids." Institute of Medicine. On healthy menu tips, check out http://www.dietaryguidelines.gov.

For a healthy sample menu, check out http://www.mypyramid.gov.

Physical Activity Guidelines for Americans, http://www.health.gov /paguidelines

Nutrition:
www.nutrition.gov
www.healthfinder.gov

Health:
www. health.gov

US Department of Agriculture (USDA)
Center for Nutrition Policy and Promotion, http://www.cnpp.usda .gov
Food and Nutrition Service, http://www.fns.usda.gov
Food and Nutrition Information Center, http://fnic.nal.usda.gov
National Institute of Food and Agriculture, http://www.nifa.usda.gov

US Department of Health and Human Services (HHS)
Office of Disease Prevention and Health Promotion, http://odphp .osophs.dhhs.gov

Food and Drug Administration, http://www.fda.gov
Centers for Disease Control and Prevention, http://www.cdc.gov
National Institutes of Health, http://www.nih.gov
Let's Move! http://www.letsmove.gov
Healthy People, http://www.healthypeople.gov
US National Physical Activity Plan, http://www.physicalactivityplan .org
American Heart Association
Institute of Medicine
Whfoods.org
Nutrient.jalaime.com
Livestrong.com

AllNigerianrecipes.com
Andrew Weil, MD, three breathing exercises
Andreoli and Carpenter's Cecil Essentials of Medicine, 8th edition
The World's Greatest Treasury of Health Secrets

Losing weight is the easy part; holding off the weight you lost is the hard part. This book will show you, step by step, how I did both. For two years and counting, it has worked for me. Now you can share in my secrets.

One of the many ways to fight back is to equip yourself with as much credible information about food as possible. My approaches were simple, practical, and successful and therefore need to be shared with the general public.

Readers will learn:

- *How I was able to lose thirty pounds and maintain it for over two years*
- *All the things I learned from my body as I went through this journey*
- *The dynamics between weight maintenance and physical fitness*
- *The relationship between obesity and diseases such as hypertension*
- *How to apply good nutrition and exercise to take control of their health*
- *To understand the basic concept of nutrition: BMR, BMI, plasticity, and cells*
- *The interaction between the brain and the gut in weight maintenance*
- *How to fight back as the food industry competes for your taste buds*
- *How I handled a two-week exercise hiatus*
- *How to fill your void with introspection rather than with food and drinks*
- *Three stages in weight-loss trajectory*
- *To make your own nature-based recipe*

Index

Page numbers in *italics* indicate figures and tables.

as macronutrient, 54–58
re-gained weight role, 86
sources of, 43, 64, 83
cardiovascular health, 20–21, 35
cell adaptation, 73–74
cerebellum, movement coordination
role, 66–68
chest pain, 70
children, eating habits of, 64, 78–
80, *78–80*
chlorothiazides, 2–3
chocolate bars, sugar in, 46–47
cigarette smoking, 81
cocoyam, 41
coffee, 5
committment, 71–73, 80, 86–87
concussions, 70
consolidation stage, of weight loss,
93
cooking tips, 81–84
coordination, 66–68
coronary artery disease, 20–21, 35
cultural behavior, obesity role, 9

D

dairy products, 33–34
desserts, avoiding, 62
diabetes, 16, 46
dietary fat
food labels and, 50
function of, 55
as macronutrient, 43, 54–58
sources of, 35–36, *43*
diets and dieting. *See* healthy habits
disease/disability, weight gain and,
11, 16–21, 70
doctors, as source of nutritional
information, 75–76

E

eating out, 10–11

ectomorph body type, 13
eddoe, 41
emotions, weight management role,
73
endomorph body type, 13
environment, for exercise, 68–69
equilibrium stage, of weight loss, 93
essential fatty acids, 56
"event-food syndrome," 9
exercise. *See* physical activity

F

facial appearance, 67–68
fast food, 12
fasting, 63
fat. *See* body fat; dietary fat
fatigue, hunger and, 63, 77
fatty acids, 35, 40, 56
fatty liver disease, 16
fiber, *42, 51*
flaxseed, 35
flu, 5
food
availability of, 8
awareness/understanding of, 75,
88–89, *90*
categories of, 31–33, *31–32,
42–43*
as companion, 8
cost of, 8–9
natural vs. processed, 32–33 (*see
also* processed foods)
rotation of types consumed, 62
food allergies, 34
food labels, 49–50
food phobias, 10
fruit, 39–41, *42–43, 51*, 97

G

gallstones, 18–19
gamma-linolenic acid, 35, 56

motivations, 86–87

movement coordination, 66–68

N

neuroplasticity, 74

night-shift work, 10

nitrosamine, 37

nonalcoholic fatty liver disease, 16

nutritional guidelines, *51*, 75–76, 99–100. *See also* healthy habits

nuts, 42, *42–43*, 43

O

oats, 38

obesity and overweight, 2, 7–13, 15–16. *See also* weight

oils, 35–36, 78

olive fruits/oil, 35

omega fatty acids, 35, 40, 56

Osgood-Schlatter disease, 70

overweight. *See* obesity and overweight

oxygenation, of blood, 17

P

palmetoleic acid, 56

pancreas, 18, 45–46

peanuts, 32, 42

peas, 84

phobias, 10

physical activity

   accessibility and equipment, 12–13, 68–69

   aging effects, 12

   calorie needs and, 27–30, *27–28*

   as priority, 11, 65–66

   thermogenesis and, *25*, 26

   weight management role, 64–69, 76–77

physical exams, 1

phytochemicals, 39, 40

plant-based diets, 64, 75–76

plant foods, edible derivatives of, 40–41, *41. See also* fruit; vegetables

plaque, arterial, 21

Pollan, Michael, 46

portion sizes, 61–62, 74

prediabetes, 16

processed foods

   avoidance of, 12, 88

   characteristics of, 33

   grain products, 38

   vs. natural foods, 32–33

   sugar in, 45, 46

protein

   in body composition, 53–54, *53*

   function of, 57

   as macronutrient, 43, 54–58

   sources of, 36–37, *43*

Q

quiz, food knowledge, *90*

R

recipe information, 81–85

relationships, as factor in weight gain, 11–12

root vegetables, 40–41

S

salt. *See* sodium

satiety, 87

saturated fats, 35–36, 50, *51*

shuffle stage, of weight loss, 93

sleep, hunger and, 63, 77

sleep apnea, 17

smoking, 81

snacking, 8, 10, 60, 77, 89

social behavior, obesity role, 9

soda, *4*, 46, *51*, 64, 88

sodium

   in foods, 34, 47–49